RUNNING ON AIR

"Over the years, I've experimented off and on with my own breathing patterns while running so I was very interested to read how Budd Coates might quantify his years of experience in print. I very much like how he has connected perceived effort with how one's breathing patterns can be consciously altered to enhance relaxation as one's pace and effort increase. He then relates this simple concept to runners at all levels by offering some very good training programs that blend his theory into a series of graded training programs that have a sound basis in exercise physiology. My advice: Give it a try for 2 months and see what happens."

—**FRANK SHORTER**, 1972 Olympic marathon gold medalist

"Women new to running will gain confidence from the simplicity and truth of Budd Coates's rhythmic breathing effort, and experienced women runners will learn how to improve, without giving more time from busy lives."

—**KATHRINE SWITZER**, women's running pioneer
and author of *Marathon Woman*

"In the 25 years that I have known and worked with Budd Coates, he has helped thousands of Rodale/*Runner's World* runners to reach their goals. *Running on Air* offers some provocative, new approaches, but all are based on a strong foundation of sound principles."

—▢▢▢, 1968 Boston Marathon winner
▢rge of *Runner's World*

"I have been research▢ and exercise performance for over 25 years. D▢ ▢hange in attitudes toward the role of breathing in p▢ my own book on breathing training for sport in 2010, I searched for books like Budd Coates's *Running on Air*— books that put breathing at the center of the coaching and training process—no such books existed. I'm delighted to see that this void has now been filled. The genius of setting training intensity using breathing effort is that this single perception integrates so many of the factors that influence one's ability to sustain a given intensity of exercise. This is the only way one can truly optimize the training stimulus, and something that a number on a heart rate monitor or GPS cannot possibly achieve."

—**ALISON K. MCCONNELL**, PhD, FACSM, FBASES,
professor of applied physiology, Brunel University, London, UK,
and author of *Breathe Strong, Perform Better*

"Budd Coates, one of America's foremost coaches, finally has written the book that runners of all levels have been waiting for. In simple, understandable language, Coates tells both mid-pack and elite runners how to improve their times while staying injury-free. Who could ask for more?"

—**GEORGE HIRSCH,** chairman of the NYRR Board
and former publisher of *Runner's World*

"Budd Coates, with expert science and the wisdom of a great coach, frees us to run naturally again, uncluttered by systems and gadgets, fueled by the air and powered by the earth."

—**ROGER ROBINSON,** senior writer, *Running Times*

"I first met Budd Coates 40 years ago when he was a skinny teen and the #3 runner on his high school's cross country team. At the time, I was the athletic director at the local YMCA, where I was just starting a radical new program: an exercise class, with running at the heart, for the average adult. Budd had talent as a runner, for sure, but he was not a natural-born superstar. However, he became a star, in fact, as a leading contender for the Olympic marathon team. He also became a star at Rodale Press, where he transforms the lives of employees—from the young to the old, the slow to the fast, and the walker to the runner. *Running on Air* now makes Budd's unique approach to training available to the world. Does Coach Bob run on air? Well, if anyone can teach an old dog new tricks, it is Budd—stay tuned. One thing is for sure, much like our mutual mentor and good friend the late Coach Bill Coughlin, Budd will give to our sport until his last breath."

—**BOB GLOVER,** author of the bestselling *The Runner's Handbook*
and *The Competitive Runner's Handbook*

"*Running on Air* by Budd Coates represents an innovative way for athletes, especially distance runners, to train and race. Rhythmic breathing requires some conscious effort at first but once learned, it becomes second nature. I especially like how Budd takes pertinent research literature and applies it to his rhythmic breathing effort scale. I highly recommend that coaches and athletes learn this breathing technique to enhance performance and potentially reduce injuries."

—**TIMOTHY J. QUINN, PHD,** exercise science option coordinator
and coordinator for graduate studies in the department
of kinesiology at the University of New Hampshire

RUNNER'S WORLD
RUNNING ON AIR

THE REVOLUTIONARY WAY TO RUN BETTER
BY **BREATHING SMARTER**

BUDD COATES, MS
AND CLAIRE KOWALCHIK

RODALE.

© 2013 by Rodale Inc.

All rights reserved. No part of this publication may be reproduced or transmitted in any form or by any means, electronic or mechanical, including photocopying, recording, or any other information storage and retrieval system, without the written permission of the publisher.

Rodale books may be purchased for business or promotional use or for special sales. For information, please write to: Special Markets Department, Rodale Inc., 733 Third Avenue, New York, NY 10017

Runner's World is a registered trademark of Rodale Inc.

Printed in the United States of America Rodale Inc. makes every effort to use acid-free ♾, recycled paper ♻.

Photographs by Thomas MacDonald/Rodale Images Illustrations © Primal Pictures Book design by Christopher Rhoads

Library of Congress Cataloging-in-Publication Data is on file with the publisher.

ISBN 978–1–60961–919–0 paperback

Distributed to the trade by Macmillan

2   4   6   8   10   9   7   5   3   1   paperback

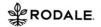

RODALE.

We inspire and enable people to improve their lives and the world around them.
rodalebooks.com

For my father, the late Morris Coates; my stepfather, the late George Hamner; and my very good friend Yoiche Furukawa.

Though you never met, your life experiences connect you. As teenagers, your first international experience was World War II, where you were forced to take the lives of others to save your own and the lives of those around you.

Some 40 years later, my first international experience was running the Fukuoka Marathon. My fight was with the marathon, and while I didn't fare too well, I did become friends with my Japanese competitors and with Yoiche. We exchanged gifts and shared the wonderful sport of running. Yo, I still remember driving your one-day-old Lincoln Continental around the streets of Ohme.

Dad, George, Yo, you never had the opportunity to share friendship, but because of running, you did share me. This book is a work of my life—a life of running that you made possible.

Contents

Foreword

"He divines remedies against injuries; he knows how to turn serious accidents to his own advantage."—Friedrich Nietzsche

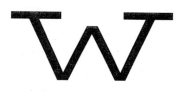ho would have thought that injuries would be the source of my success as a runner? Who could have foreseen that injuries would be what cracked the door, opening the way for me to discover a new vision of training and racing that would lead me to become a four-time qualifier for the US Olympic Marathon Trials, race a 2:13 personal best for the marathon, and enjoy a streak of 13 wins at the annual 3.5-mile JPMorgan Chase & Co. Corporate Challenge in New York City? But that is the way it happened.

Like many runners, I took up the sport in high school—for me, that was back in the '70s—and as a senior on the cross-country team, I won the individual league championship, a good but not great accomplishment. I continued to run at Springfield College in Massachusetts, where

I majored in physical education. At the college level, cross-country races jump from the 5-K of high school to 8-K and 10-K, and the racing schedule gets rigorous. We raced often with little time to recover, and as a consequence, I was injured often. Consistency in training is vital to a runner's success. When injury constantly forces you to take time off, you lose a lot of quality training time. As renowned coach and exercise physiologist Jack Daniels puts it, "It's easier to stay fit than get fit."

I spent lots of time in the college's physiology building (there were no cross-training facilities for athletes then) on a Monarch test bike, pedaling away to maintain my conditioning when I couldn't run. After my cycling sessions, Dr. A.J. "Jack" Mahurin would suggest a book for me to read. First he recommended *Running the Lydiard Way* by Arthur Lydiard and Garth Gilmour, then *Stress* by Hans Selye, and after that *The Van-Aaken Method* by Ernst VanAaken. These books significantly influenced my training, helping me to stay healthy and to improve as a runner, and I continue to follow much of their advice today. But in 1976, they did not resolve my recurring injuries.

I continued to dig through the exercise research and eventually came across an article by Ian Jackson called "Breath Play" that found a relationship between breathing cycles and running cadence. Later I found a study by Dennis Bramble, PhD, and David Carrier, PhD, of the University of Utah, explaining that the greatest impact stress of running occurs when one's footstrike coincides with the beginning of an exhalation. This means, for example, that if you begin to exhale every time your left foot hits the ground, the left side of your body will continually suffer the greatest running stress, making it more vulnerable to injury.

Hmm. My most frequent injury was to my *left* hip flexor. So I began to think, what if I could create a pattern that coordinated footstrike and breathing such that I would land alternately on my left foot and then my right foot at the beginning of every exhale? This would distribute the impact stress of running equally across both sides of my body and then, perhaps, I could finally get healthy. It was worth a try.

I developed a pattern of rhythmic breathing that I adapted to all aspects of my running and began using it between my junior and senior years of college. I ran well enough my senior year to earn my one and only varsity letter. I also trained for and ran my first marathon the winter before graduating from Springfield and finished in a respectable 2:52:45. With these results, I knew I was on to something.

I continued to work on a rhythmic breathing method of running while pursuing my master's degree in physical education and exercise physiology at Illinois State University, during which time I trained for my second marathon. I continued to apply rhythmic breathing to my running, but I homed in on a five-step pattern for easy training and a three-step cycle for faster running. I used the three-step pattern during that second marathon and ran an incredibly even 2:33:29.

I tested the method out again in 1981 at the Boston Marathon. I was working at Rodale Inc., where I continue to work today, as director of corporate fitness. One of my very good friends at Rodale, Pat Corpora, had run Boston a few times with great success but wanted to break 2:40. The barrier, as I saw it, was that he always went out a bit too fast, as we've all done. Pat and I agreed to run together at least for the first half of the race, and I would help him run under control. We ran that first 13 miles using a five-step rhythmic breathing pattern and came through the halfway point in 79 minutes—just right. Then I picked up my pace and my rhythmic breathing to the three-step pattern and completed the second half in 67 minutes (2:26) while Pat finished in 2:35:48. Both of us had raced to PRs. That experience convinced me that I could manage my effort through rhythmic breathing with a great deal of success.

I spent the next 30 years fine-tuning my rhythmic breathing method, continuing to dig through all the research I could find on breathing and exercise, using rhythmic breathing in my training and racing, and I've enjoyed many personal successes. In addition to the accomplishments I mentioned earlier, I've won marathons in the US and internationally, and

I've run sub-3-hour marathons in five different decades—something fewer than 30 people in the world have achieved.

It is my job but also among my personal values to share what I know or have learned about healthy living, exercise, fitness, and, of course, running with others. At Rodale and within my local community, I've coached a number of distance runners to personal bests, as well as qualifying times for the Boston Marathon and the US Olympic Marathon Trials. In addition, I've taught thousands of beginning runners and helped them to reach their goals and develop a love for running that I believe they'll carry with them for a lifetime. Though I began writing this book about 2 years ago, in truth it has been more than 30 years in the making. I hope *Running on Air* helps you reach your goals, whatever they may be, and helps you love running as much as I do.

—*Budd Coates*

Preface

I t was the best piece of running advice anyone ever gave me: "Leave your watch at home."

I had been using Budd's training schedules to prepare for races but had asked for little training advice. I was working as an editor at *Runner's World* magazine at the time, and I'd apply whatever piece of strategy was pressed upon me by whichever talented athlete I had come to know. Most of those tips had to do with running more miles and running them faster. And they didn't work. My race times slowed and my race experiences turned into struggles from start to finish.

I was complaining to Budd, telling him I was ready to give up racing altogether. Let's face it, I thought, I'm not athletic anyway. I didn't participate in sports growing up, because I simply couldn't. I can still feel the sting of humiliation from that day on the playground when my fifth-grade teacher helped me swing the bat during a softball game so that I'd be able to make contact. Yes, I was one of those nerds picked last or near to last for any team in PE. So what was I thinking? Racing? Really?

"Leave your watch at home," Budd said. "On the days when you feel good, you'll naturally run faster, and when you're fatigued, you'll run slower, which is what you should do. You'll run according to how your body feels on that day."

I tried it and, in combination with the training schedules Budd wrote for me, it worked. I ran PR after PR at every distance. I dropped my 5-K finishes from 27 minutes to just over 21. My 10-Ks fell from 56 minutes to 42. I even won the women's division of a local 10-K. I qualified for and ran the Boston Marathon, racing negative splits (second half faster than the first), and crossed the finish line in 3:36 (and that was before race chips). Budd even coached me to a 5:58 for a 1-mile road race.

I loved it—the training, the racing, the PRs. But perhaps what mattered most to me, and still does, was that the little girl who couldn't hit a softball, make a basket, or kick a soccer ball down the field had become an athlete. So 20 years later, when Budd asked if I would help him write this book, I answered with a resounding yes.

Looking back, I see that Budd's advice to leave my watch at home was the kernel of a greater training philosophy, one that underpins the unique method of running, training, and racing presented in this book. Those many years ago, Budd had introduced me to the count patterns of rhythmic breathing that you will soon discover. Happily—and surprisingly—I fell into them naturally. But those patterns are simply the framework of a way of running that goes much deeper, a method that is so very simple yet so very full of substance and so broad in application. It's a method drawn from physiology and that draws on your own unique physiology, a method that reaches back to the wisdom of some of our sport's most masterful coaches and brings that wisdom forward, refining it for today's runner.

This is running in its purest form. No heart monitors, no watches, no GPS. Just you. Running in rhythm with your body. Running from within. Running in synchronicity with the effort of the moment. And this is precisely why the rhythmic breathing training method works. This way of running will take you to your fastest performances and your most pleasurable runs. It will lead you, if you choose to follow, to a lifetime of running at its best.

I know this to be true. Today, more than 20 years after first leaving my watch at home and many miles past my best performances, I still lace up my running shoes, head out the door, and, though my pace is much slower, I continue to run not against the clock but *with* my body. It feels exactly the same. It's everything I love about running that keeps me running. Me, moving over the earth. Footsteps, breaths rhythmically sounding. Air filling my lungs. Perfect.

—*Claire Kowalchik*

CHAPTER 1

RUN STRONGER, LONGER, FASTER

"My conversion to a rhythmic runner over 30 years ago and its positive effect on my mostly injury-free status as a runner allowed me to progress from a filler on my college cross-country team to a four-time qualifier for the US Olympic Marathon Trials." —Budd Coates

Whether you're a beginning, intermediate, or elite runner, each of us has a running goal. Perhaps it's to establish a weekly running routine for fitness, or to run a 5-K, half-marathon, or marathon, or to compete at the sport's highest level. To achieve any of those goals, a runner needs to be able to run consistently from week to week. It's not so much exactly *what* you do in training but the fact that you are able to maintain your training over a long period that allows you to run farther and faster.

Rhythmic breathing can play a key role in keeping you injury-free, as it has done for me. But to understand how that can happen, let's first take a look at some of the stresses of running. When your foot hits the ground, the force of impact equals two to three times your body weight. Research by Dennis Bramble, PhD, and David Carrier, PhD, of the University of Utah shows that the impact stress is greatest when footstrike coincides with the beginning of an exhalation.

Another factor in the impact-injury equation is this: When you exhale, your diaphragm and the muscles associated with the diaphragm relax, creating less stability in your core and making you more susceptible to injury. When you combine these two factors, your foot strikes the ground at the beginning of exhalation, when impact stress is the greatest and core stability is lowest. It's the perfect storm for injury.

TRY THIS: Get up and walk around. Pay attention to your breathing and footsteps, and notice those points when your foot hits the ground as you begin to exhale—those are the moments of greatest impact stress, whether you are walking or running.

Now let's consider one more variable. Let's say that when you run, you always land on your right foot at the beginning of each exhalation. The right side of your body will continuously suffer the greatest impact force of running, becoming increasingly worn down and vulnerable to injury. If your left foot strikes the ground with the beginning of every exhale, the left side of your body will become susceptible to injury, as was my experience.

Rhythmic breathing coordinates footstrike with inhalation and exhalation in an odd/even pattern so that you will land alternately on your right and left foot at the beginning of every exhalation. This way, the impact stress of running will be shared equally across both sides of your body.

An analogy would be if you loaded a backpack down with books, notebooks, and a laptop and then slung it over your right shoulder. With all this weight on one side of your body, you'd be forced to compensate physically, placing more stress on one side of your back and hip. But if you were to slip that same heavy backpack over both shoulders, the load would be distributed evenly. That way, you put your body in a position to better manage that stress and your back stays healthy.

Rhythmic breathing achieves in the day-to-day microcosm of running what rhythmic training (a pattern of hard/easy training) accomplishes in the macrocosm. If you run hard day after day with no letup, you *will* become injured. Any form of exercise stresses the body. You need to give your muscles and bones time to bounce back before applying that

Ditch the Stitches

Stitches, side-stickers, whatever you want to call them, we've all experienced those annoying sharp little pains that jab the side of your torso and can stop you in your tracks, even if only temporarily. You've likely read a dozen different techniques for relieving them. Become a rhythmic runner and you can avoid them altogether.

Swedish exercise physiologist Finn Rost offered the theory that when the diaphragm moves upward during exhalation and organs drop down during footstrike, the tension created forces the diaphragm into spasm. Owen Anderson, PhD, author of *The Science of Running,* supports this, saying, "Since the diaphragm is in the up position when you are breathing out . . . stitch chances are maximized when footstrike and exhalation are synchronized on one side of the body."

Most runners who run with an even 2/2 breathing pattern (inhale for two steps/exhale for two steps) exhale consistently on the right footstrike. And interestingly, studies show that the majority of runners experience stitches on their right side.

Rhythmic breathing uses an odd/even pattern so that exhalation and footstrike are *not* synchronized on one side of the body but instead alternate from right to left. In addition, rhythmic breathing creates a rhythm of contraction and relaxation in the muscles used in breathing, helping them to work more efficiently. This combination of the effects of rhythmic breathing will allow you to run stitch-free. That's what runner Leah Zerbe has found. You can read her story on page 68.

stress again. A relentless regimen of hard running leaves no time for recovery from the work—it tears you down until you suffer an injury. Therefore, it stands to reason that if one side of the body relentlessly endures the greatest impact stress, that side will become worn down and vulnerable to injury. Rhythmic breathing—again, in the microcosm—allows both sides of the body a slight rest from the greatest immediate impact stress of running.

But there's more to rhythmic breathing than a pattern of footstrikes, exhales, and inhales that keeps you injury-free. Rhythmic breathing focuses your attention on your breath and opens the way for breathing to become the source of how you train and race.

Mind/Body Training

Years ago, famed coaching pioneers, including Ernst Van Aaken, Percy Cerutty, Arthur Lydiard, and Mihaly Igloi, designed training programs using effort levels that were determined and described not by scientific measurement but by perception. Lydiard, for example, would define effort in fractions—½, ¾, whole. Igloi would reference easy, good, fresh, hard, very hard, and all-out efforts. And those efforts were "measured" by how hard an athlete was breathing and how hard the athlete was working. How fast or hard did the effort *feel*?

Once scientists—exercise physiologists—began to study training and its relationship to the body, the emphasis shifted from breathing to the cardiovascular system. Their attention focused on heart rate, pumping volume, and how energy production in working muscles translated to performance. Exercise physiologists convinced coaches and athletes that these responses to running were the key measurable components of any successful training program. The thinking was that because these elements could be measured, training could be made more scientific, more exact, and therefore more effective.

Workouts were defined around effort as a percentage of maximum heart rate; therefore, measuring heart rate became the definitive training tool for runners. And here's how that worked: You would stop running, quickly find your pulse, glance at your stopwatch, count, and then calculate beats per minute to determine the percentage of maximum heart rate at which you were running. It was "scientific training" even if terribly inaccurate. Once heart rate monitors came along, this method became much more accurate—and expensive. But it turned running into a machine/body experience. Runners set their pace according to a number on a display, not according to how they felt. Running succeeds best at all levels when it is a mind/body experience. The need to breathe deeper and faster during running increases much the same as the need for your heart to fill deeper and beat faster, but it is much easier (and gadget-free) to monitor your breathing than it is to monitor your heart rate. And it is direct and immediate. A heart rate monitor is a "middle man" in your training, so to speak. It picks up signals from your cardiovascular system and then shares them with you. By focusing on your breathing, *you* pick up the signals—you *feel* the effort.

Swimmers have been training this way for years. Bob Timmons, who coached Jim Ryun—the first high school runner to break 4 minutes in the mile—was quoted as saying that runners could learn a lot from the way swimmers train. When it comes to breathing, he was right.

But what about the numbers? you ask. *The heart rate monitor gives me numbers to follow; how will I know if my breathing rate is where it is supposed to be for any given workout?* Good question. I have developed a simple system and scale that combine rhythmic breathing with perceived exertion so that it will be easy for you to know what your level of effort is at any point during a run. This system will be explained in detail later in the book. Suffice it to say for now that this rhythmic breathing method combines the best of both worlds—it relies on the simplicity of the mind/body connection to provide instant feedback along with a scale of measurement to identify your level of running effort. This becomes invaluable during racing, especially as you explode off the starting line.

Mind/Body Racing

You may have experienced moments running or racing when you've "lost your breath," or feel like you need to "catch your breath," or you're waiting for your "second wind." Here's what's happening on a very simplified physiological level. Your muscles need oxygen to perform the work you are asking them to do—run—and as your muscles use oxygen, they produce carbon dioxide (a by-product of metabolism). You breathe air into your lungs. Oxygen diffuses into your bloodstream, and your circulatory system delivers that oxygen to your working muscles, where, in exchange, it picks up the unwanted carbon dioxide. Blood flows back to the lungs to release the carbon dioxide and pick up more oxygen for your busy muscles.

The more work your muscles do, the more oxygen they burn and the more carbon dioxide (CO_2) they produce, which diffuses back into the bloodstream and is carried to the lungs. The catch is that the need for more oxygen (O_2) is immediate but the response to that need isn't. Excess carbon dioxide in the bloodstream is the signal to your brain that more oxygen is needed. Not until that excess CO_2 is delivered back to the lungs is the message picked up by your central nervous system, which then triggers faster and deeper breathing in an effort to replace the CO_2 leaving your blood with oxygen. This lag creates a period in which you don't have enough oxygen for the work you are doing. That, coupled with the fact that you may be working at an effort above which you can supply the necessary O_2, creates an oxygen debt. You're running anaerobically and you've lost your breath. At this point you have three options: Stop running, continue running to the point of total fatigue (which won't be much longer), or slow way down. Most of us choose option three.

As your running slows, so does the work your muscles are doing. The increase in your breathing gradually supplies enough oxygen to your fatiguing, less active muscles. At the same time, your muscles produce less CO_2, signaling the brain that less oxygen is needed, and breathing relaxes. Once you've recovered from this burst off the starting line, you can then pick up your pace to a manageable level and settle into a breathing rhythm that you can maintain over the remaining miles. You've "caught your breath" or "found your second wind"—you are now running aerobically. Glenn Town, PhD, an exercise physiologist at Westmont College in Santa Barbara, California, refers to this as "catching up." You have, however, lost valuable time dealing with that near shutdown of your body.

A runner experienced in rhythmic breathing can avoid this altogether. The rhythmic runner has developed a mind/body awareness of the connections between pace, effort, and breathing. She can increase pace while monitoring the effort through the need to breathe faster. When the work of running corresponds to the appropriate level on the Rhythmic Breathing Effort Scale (see Chapter 4), the runner settles into that pace and wastes no time recovering from an overzealous start. Long before reaching the 1-mile digital clock in a race, the rhythmic breather knows she is on pace and at the right level of effort.

Rhythmic breathing can also be used to advantage in racing strategically. As Frank Shorter, the 1972 Olympic gold medalist in the marathon, puts it, "Races typically take place in surges—hard efforts alternating with bouts of recovery. The winners aren't necessarily the fastest runners, they're the ones who can recover from the surges the fastest."

Relief from Asthma

You know how the environment can impact your running. For the asthma sufferer, that impact can be magnified to an unbearable level. Exercise-induced asthma is, in short, an adverse reaction of the lungs and breathing muscles to a sudden change in breathing patterns, but it can also be triggered or exacerbated by cold air, high pollen counts, or other environmental factors. The alveoli—small air sacs in the lungs where the exchange of oxygen and carbon dioxide takes place—become constricted and the breathing muscles respond with rapid, erratic contractions. Rhythmic breathing may reduce or even eliminate exercise-induced asthma in runners because it fosters a calm, smooth increase in breathing rate and depth. Read how one runner used rhythmic breathing to help ease his exercise-induced asthma on page 9.

Rhythmic breathing helps you to gauge these surges—both yours and your competitors'—and prevents you from overstepping your level of fitness so that you can race as efficiently as possible. It gives you seamless control over your racing from start to finish.

A Lifetime of Running

Not only will rhythmic breathing help keep you injury-free for a lifetime of running and racing, but the mind/body pattern of breathing and running that is individually yours will last a lifetime.

A great friend and former running partner of mine, Mark Will-Weber, author of *The Quotable Runner*, asked me not too long ago if I was still doing long runs and hard workouts. I said yes, just not as fast. I am still running at the same rhythmic breathing levels as I did when I was in my twenties. I have a 22-mile hill run that I call my Waiatarua Circuit. (The Waiatarua Circuit is a 22-mile training course laid out by legendary coach Arthur Lydiard over the hills around Auckland, New Zealand. It ranges over a series of hills, including one 3 miles in length.) When I run this loop in preparation for a marathon, I can check my watch at the top of the last hill and see within 1 to 2 minutes what my marathon time will be. And it's held true for 30 years.

Rhythmic Runner:
Logan Blyler

RUNNER PROFILE: competitive runner in high school, college, and postcollege

AGE: 23

OCCUPATION: athletic director (middle and high school), Eastern University Academy Charter School

> "These were drastic changes in my race times, and the only difference was that I was using rhythmic breathing."

It was a warm spring day for the high school track meet in Nazareth, Pennsylvania. Logan Blyler was getting ready to start his kick at the end of his leg in the 4 X 800 relay when his foot caught with another runner and he went down. He couldn't catch his breath and fell into an asthma attack. Blyler had suffered from exercise-induced asthma (caused by abrupt changes to breathing) as a child but thought he had grown out of it.

Often, it takes a fall to push you to your highest potential.

Budd Coates, whose daughter, Kelsey, also ran high school track, happened to be at that meet. Days later he invited Blyler to dis-

cuss rhythmic breathing and its potential for managing asthma. "We had a lengthy meeting," Blyler recalls. "It made sense that controlled breathing could help me control my asthma during abrupt changes in speed, so I decided to give it a try." And it worked. In the 7 years that Blyler has been using rhythmic breathing, he hasn't experienced a single asthma attack.

Blyler discovered other benefits of this new way of breathing as well. "I had been struggling with improving my race times. I could not break through," he says. "Then, within 1 year of putting it [rhythmic breathing] into place, my mile dropped from the 4:50s to the low 4:40s. In cross-country, I had been stuck in the upper 17s [for the 5-K] and brought that time down to the lower 17s.

"I had always been consistent with my training. I always pushed when I raced," Blyler continues. "These were drastic changes in my race times, and the only difference was that I was using rhythmic breathing."

When Blyler plunged into college cross-country, where distances jump up to 8-K and 10-K and the race schedule is relentless, rhythmic breathing again proved a key asset. "Because I could pace myself and control my breathing, I could prevent getting worn out, and it gave me a step ahead of some of the other athletes who may have had more talent," he explains.

Now a coach, Blyler teaches rhythmic breathing to his middle school and high school runners.

"You can use it to control how you respond—when your muscles start tensing up and you begin to breathe more frantically, you can slow down your breathing without changing your pace," he explains. "It gives you more control over how much oxygen goes into your system. You use energy more efficiently, which allows you to work harder in the latter part of a distance event."

And Blyler's athletes have enjoyed the results. His mid-distance runners use rhythmic breathing to keep a consistent pace, and even his sprinters have harnessed the steady rhythm to achieve successful results, with one athlete slashing his 100-meter times from 11.04 to under 10.8.

The results are in and will continue to come in, but Blyler needs no more convincing that rhythmic breathing works.

CHAPTER 2

THE SWEET SPOT

"By rhythmical breathing one may bring himself into harmonious vibration with nature."

—Yogi Ramacharaka, pseud. William Atkinson

The year was 1970. The place was Camden, New York. I was in eighth grade, about to start a spring baseball practice. Our team was acting a bit rowdy and our coach, Coach Davis, decided to calm us down by ordering us to run some laps around the gymnasium. Four laps into this "punishment," I mentally drifted into a zone and found myself enjoying it. It was my first-ever "sweet spot," where running seems effortless and you feel like you could go on forever. And what takes me back to that place—that feeling—today, over and over again, is rhythmic breathing.

Breath Awareness

Attention to breathing has a long history in Eastern philosophy. Dennis Lewis, a longtime student of Taoism and other Eastern philosophies, teaches breathing and leads workshops throughout the US at venues including the Esalen Institute and the Kripalu Center for Yoga and Health. In his book *The Tao of Natural Breathing*, Lewis shares the following Taoist belief: "To breathe fully is to live fully, to manifest the full range of power of our inborn potential for vitality in everything that we sense, feel, think, and do." In Hinduism, yoga teaches pranayama—breath work. *Prana* means breath as a life-giving force: The work of breathing draws life-giving force into the body. And that work is accomplished through diaphragmatic breathing, which means that as you inhale, you contract the diaphragm fully to allow maximum volume in the thoracic (chest) cavity for maximum expansion of the lungs and maximum intake of air. Rhythmic breathing does the same, drawing the breath—the life force—into the body through controlled, focused diaphragmatic breathing. Through rhythmic running we breathe fully and, as the Taoists would say, realize our vitality.

Rhythmic breathing also creates a pathway to a deep centeredness. Practitioners of every style of yoga, martial arts, relaxation, and meditation use breath work to connect mind, body, and spirit. In the martial arts, this inner connection and centeredness allows more immediate and precise control of the physical body.

The same can be accomplished in running through rhythmic breathing. You achieve centeredness first by focusing your mind on fitting your breathing to an optimal footstrike pattern. Then your awareness of breathing links mind and body and creates a smooth pathway to gauging the effort of running. Rhythmic breathing helps you to *feel* your running, and that ability to feel your running allows you immediate and precise control.

"Yoga teaches that controlling your breathing can help you control your body and quiet your mind," say experts at the Mayo Clinic. When we allow ourselves to become distracted by trying to match our running effort to a pace we've defined with numbers on a watch, we break that mind/body connection. We open up a gap where stress and tension can enter and eventually wear us down. And we create a disturbance in the flow of running that hinders our success and enjoyment. Rhythmic breathing in and of itself is calming, and awareness of breathing draws your focus toward calm. It allows you to remain as relaxed as possible, quieting any stress in the body that could inhibit performance. And if you should feel a twinge of tension or discomfort,

Training in the Sweet Spot

You can achieve a meditative state while running at any pace—even race pace—but if you are training to compete and are following a pattern of hard, moderate, and easy workouts, you'll find that the meditative run best suits your moderate or long run. During that run—which will feel effortless—your thoughts will drift away from the physical work, so you will need to occasionally "check in" with your body to make sure you are running at the appropriate effort for that workout.

The rhythmic breathing effort that brings me into the meditative zone is a 51-52 on the Rhythmic Breathing Effort Scale, which I will explain in detail in Chapter 4. The effort is easy but not my easiest. When I'm running over slightly hilly terrain, my physical rhythm and pace will stay the same, but my breathing effort will increase just a bit on the inclines. Because I am in "the zone" and my thoughts are wandering, I sometimes don't notice that I've sneaked into this higher effort of running and maintained it beyond the incline when it should drop back to an easier pace and effort. You may find, too, that fluctuations in the environment will push your effort to a level that is just a bit too hard for the workout you are meant to do. Working harder than what is appropriate can add to your fatigue and slow your recovery. Remember, every workout has a purpose.

you can mentally "push" it out of the body as you exhale. Ironically, being in tune with your body's effort through breathing allows you to run effortlessly.

Being in Rhythm

"Rhythm pervades the universe," writes Yogi Ramacharaka (aka William Atkinson) in his book *Science of Breath.* "The swing of the planets around the sun; the rise and fall of the sea; the beating of the heart; the ebb and flow of the tide; all follow rhythmic laws. Our bodies are as much subject to rhythmic laws as is the planet in its revolution around the sun."

Through running the body falls into rhythm—the rhythmic stepping of our feet, beating of our heart, inhalation and exhalation of our breath.

"The rhythm produced by the Yogi breath," says Atkinson, "is such as to bring the whole system, including the brain, under perfect control, and in perfect harmony." And this, he tells us, is the perfect condition for a spiritual connection to the world around us.

The synchronized cadence of running and rhythmic breathing also creates the perfect condition for us to achieve an inner connection with the world. It allows us to drift into a state of meditation that links us with our surroundings and separates us from the labor of physical work. In this state, also referred to as "the zone" or "the sweet spot," your mind and body blend together rhythmically, seamlessly, so you don't have to consciously think about what you're doing. Running just happens, easily, smoothly, comfortably. Your thoughts are free to wander as your body carries you smoothly down the road or over the trail. You feel as though you could run forever.

Sakyong Mipham knows this feeling. Mipham is the leader of Shambhala, a worldwide community of meditation and retreat centers, and an accomplished runner who has completed nine marathons. In his book *Running with the Mind of Meditation*, Mipham emphasizes that to achieve a meditative state during running, we must start with the breath. "Being with the breath is the most effective way of being in the present," he explains. "When we've established the ability to pay attention to the breath, our ability to focus on any other object or endeavor is strengthened." He adds that when we focus on our breathing and "pace" our breathing, we develop a rhythmic flow in and out, which calms the mind.

The patterned breathing that you will learn in this book has the same effect of bringing you into the present, connecting body and mind and freeing you from outside distractions. Again, as Mipham describes, "You will become more aware of your internal environment—your rhythm, the pounding of your heart, your feet hitting the trail. At the same time, you tune into your external environment—the sky, the air, the sounds of life." Mipham refers to this as *panoramic awareness*. "When the mind is totally present, it is relaxed, nimble, and sensitive. It feels lighter and clearer. It notices everything but is not distracted by anything. It is the feeling of knowing exactly where you are and what you are doing."

For me, during moderate or long runs, rhythmic breathing allows me to slide easily into an effort and pace at which everything glides on auto-pilot. My breathing is comfortable, my cadence is smooth and even, and the rhythm of both combines for that "harmonious vibration with nature."

Rhythmic Runner:
Robyn Jasko

RUNNER PROFILE: runs 20 to 25 miles a week for fitness "and to keep my sanity!"; has raced 5-K, half-marathon, and marathon

AGE: 34

OCCUPATION: creative services director, consumer magazines

> "It's meditative to use rhythmic breathing while running. Once I get in the groove, I just motor along. And I don't ever get out of breath."

Robyn Jasko was working out in the gym when she overheard a fellow runner rave about Budd Coates's rhythmic breathing method, so she decided to give it a try. "After a few runs I noticed that my pace had increased by a full minute, from 10-minute miles to 9-minute miles, without putting in much more effort," she says. "I was so excited. I had been trying to break that time barrier for years, and rhythmic breathing made it happen."

Breaking barriers and running faster are loads of fun for Jasko— "I love that I can shift into a faster run by switching from the 3:2 to the 2:1 breathing pattern," she says—but balance best describes her running goals, and rhythmic breathing gets her there.

"I've been using rhythmic breathing for about 2 years, and it's become a natural part of my running. I even find myself doing it while walking or on the elliptical trainer," she says. "It keeps me steady, balanced, and well-paced.

"It's even meditative," Jasko adds. "Once I get in the groove, I just motor along. And I don't ever get out of breath."

And Jasko doesn't ever want to stop running. "Running is like breathing to me," she says. "It's just something that I do. My goal is to keep running. I want to focus on staying injury-free and enjoying my runs, not chase a set time. I know rhythmic breathing will help me stay healthy and allow me to continue to enjoy the balanced, meditative side of running."

CHAPTER 3

THE SCIENCE OF BREATHING

"Man may exist some time without eating; a shorter time without drinking; but without breathing his existence may be measured by a few minutes."

—Yogi Ramacharaka, pseud. William Atkinson, *Science of Breath*

D ay in, day out, we breathe unaware. Awake, asleep, we inhale and exhale, continuously, regularly. Breathing is a constant. It is automatic. We take it for granted until an upper respiratory infection or asthma or even intense exertion calls our attention to it. Then we can't get our mind off breathing. Why? Because we need to breathe to live, and also because we do have some control over our breathing. The yogis are correct to say that breath is a life-giving force. It is essential to the energy-production cycle that feeds our brain and other organs and fuels our muscles for work—for running. Understanding the mechanisms of breathing can help any runner, from beginner to elite, learn to harness this force for easier, stronger, faster running.

The Mechanics

As you sit reading this book, you're breathing. You inhale. Air enters your nose and travels to your lungs. Oxygen from the air diffuses into your blood and is transported to working organs and muscles. You exhale. That is breathing from the most simplistic view. Let's look a little closer.

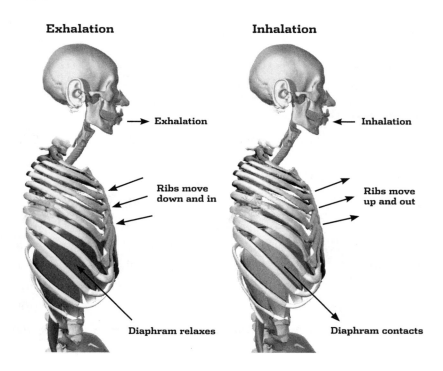

An Evolution
of Breathing

Back in 1978, Bob Glover, author, runner, coach, and friend, wrote *The Runner's Handbook*. In it, he covered breathing in four short paragraphs. Bob is a no-nonsense guy and believed that runners should breathe from their bellies, but other than that he advised that you should simply "breathe when you feel like breathing." He expanded a bit on that in his 1985 revision of *The Runner's Handbook* by adding that "some runners enjoy breathing in tune to their footstrike." By 1999, Bob acknowledged an even greater connection between running and breathing, discussing it over three pages of *The Competitive Runner's Handbook*, which includes this passage: "Most runners breathe in time with their footsteps, whether they realize it or not. We tend to breathe in a footed pattern, breathing in and out when landing on a particular foot. Most runners are right-footed breathers, inhaling and exhaling off the right foot." Bob's observations about breathing patterns during running bring us to the point today where we can look at those patterns, see how they affect running performance, and learn how to adjust them for our best performance, whether the goal is pleasurable fitness running or to compete at our highest potential. Thomas S. Miller, PhD, the author of *Programmed to Run* (2002), includes breathing skills in his chapter on stride mechanics. Miller discusses his belief that "attention to breathing" can improve efficiency and performance, and his doctoral work supported that thought.

Beneath your lungs lies the diaphragm. When you inhale, the diaphragm contracts, moving downward toward your belly button. In addition, the external intercostal muscles of your chest contract to pull your rib cage up and out. These two actions open up space or volume in your thoracic (chest) cavity. This increased space lowers the air pressure in your chest relative to the air outside your body. By the laws of physics, air moves from a place of higher pressure to an area of lower pressure, and so air is drawn into your lungs. During exhalation, the diaphragm and external intercostal muscles relax, the space in your thoracic cavity gets smaller, and air is pushed out.

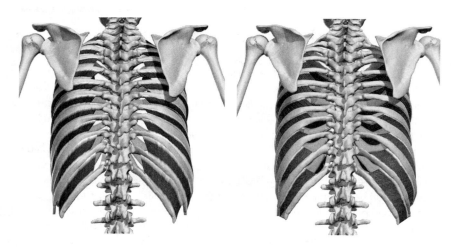

Muscles that assist in forceful exhalations as the diaphragm and external intercostal muscles (as shown) relax.

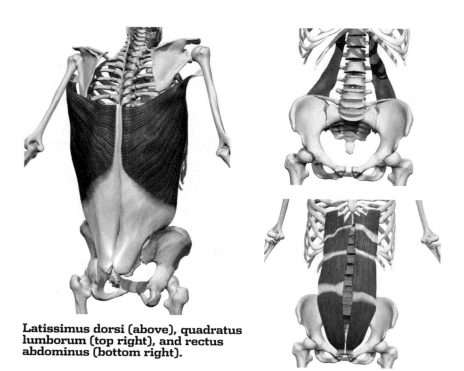

Latissimus dorsi (above), quadratus lumborum (top right), and rectus abdominus (bottom right).

When exercise requires you to breathe faster and deeper, the diaphragm works harder and additional muscles outside the chest cavity (scalene, sternocleidomastoid, and pectorals) join in to expand the thoracic cavity during inhalation. On the exhale, the internal intercostal muscles, latissimus dorsi and quadratus lumborum, combine with the rectus abdominus to forcefully push air out of the lungs. Think of a bellows—you open up the bellows to draw air in, and push it together to force air out.

The Control Center

As you've been reading this book, have you been consciously contracting your muscles to inhale and then relaxing them as you exhale? No. Breathing, like the beating of the heart, is an involuntary action. Your brain automatically takes care of this for you, regularly and continuously sending signals to your respiratory system to trigger breathing. How does your brain know when to send the signal to breathe? It does so in response to how much carbon dioxide (CO_2) is in your blood.

TRY THIS: While sitting still, continue to breathe normally for approximately 30 seconds.

- Now gradually and comfortably breathe more deeply for 30 seconds.

- Return to normal breathing.

- Next, breathe more shallowly (quick but calm) for 30 seconds.

- Return to normal breathing.

- Now force a quick breath out and suck a quick breath in.

- For the next 30 seconds, try to slow down or speed up your heart rate—while sitting still.

Which can you control quickly and easily—your heart rate or your breathing?

The purpose of breathing is to gather oxygen for your working organs and muscles, where it is used to burn glucose (blood sugar), fat, and protein to produce energy. Oxygen from the air in your lungs diffuses into your bloodstream and is transported to your organs and muscles. As your muscles work, they produce CO_2, which diffuses into the blood and is transported eventually back to the lungs. There, CO_2 diffuses into the lungs and oxygen enters the blood for the return trip to the muscles and organs. This is known as the oxygen/carbon exchange.

The harder your muscles work, the more CO_2 they produce that then gets shipped to your lungs. Rising CO_2 levels in the blood are a signal to your brain that more oxygen is needed. Your brain (the medulla oblongata in particular), in turn, signals your respiratory muscles to work harder so that more oxygen can be delivered. You begin to breathe deeper and/or faster to increase the amount of oxygen-carrying air into your lungs. And all of this happens without you giving it a thought.

Your heart also responds to a greater workload by increasing the volume of blood it pumps and beating faster so that circulating blood

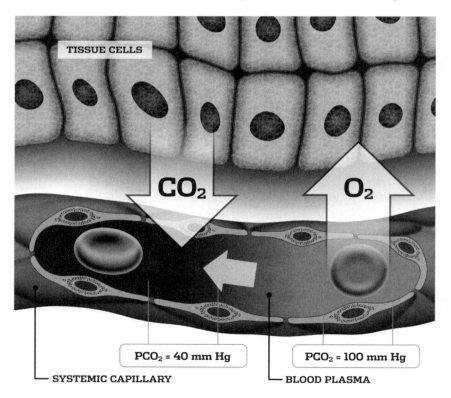

The pathways of the oxygen and carbon dioxide exchange between the working muscle and bloodstream during breathing.

can quickly deliver more food and oxygen to organs and muscles. But unlike your heartbeat, which you can't control with direct thought, you *can* change the way you breathe. You can breathe faster, slower, more deeply, more shallowly. You can breathe through your nose, through your mouth, or both. You can breathe to a certain rhythm: for example, inhale for three beats and then exhale for three beats. Breathing is an involuntary action, and it is also a *voluntary* one that can be directed by a different area of the brain called the cortex. This is the secret to how breathing can be an effective tool to help you run smarter, stronger, and faster.

Breathing and Running

Let's apply everything we've learned about breathing to the run. You walk out the door of your house and you're relaxed, breathing slowly, shallowly. You begin to run comfortably. Your muscles are working harder and producing more CO_2, which is transported through your bloodstream to your lungs, where it is traded for some oxygen. Your brain receives the word that CO_2 has increased and more oxygen is needed. The brain signals your respiratory center to breathe faster and deeper to bring more air into the lungs. Your circulatory system gets the message that it needs to pick up the pace of delivery of oxygen and fuel. Blood volume increases and your heart beats harder and faster. Soon breathing and circulation are working at a higher level and delivering what's needed to your working muscles. This has all happened automatically, and you run comfortably down the road.

Then you come upon a steep hill. The intensity of work rises sharply, and lots of CO_2 is produced by your working muscles. Your blood carries that load of CO_2 to your lungs, but the amount of oxygen available is only at the level that was required when you were running comfortably on flat ground, so your blood heads back to your muscles with less oxygen than is needed. Remember, it's the amount of CO_2 in your blood that is the signal to the brain that breathing needs to increase. As work increases, there is a lag between the need for oxygen and the delivery.

Ah, but you now know that you don't have to leave this process entirely up to the automatic nature of controlled breathing. You can choose to breathe deeper and faster, and though you cannot store oxygen in your lungs, you can cut the lag time. But how do you determine when to increase breathing and how fast or deeply to breathe? You first need to learn to judge your efforts, using breathing as a gauge, over a variety of terrains and environmental conditions. I'll show you how to do that a little later in this book.

An Overlooked Art

Exercise physiologists have long shied away from considering the idea that runners and coaches could use breathing as a tool for better training and racing. In the '60s and '70s, as scientists monitored the body's response to exercise, they discovered max VO_2—a measurement of your ability to take in oxygen and use it. Max VO_2 was thought to be the most important indicator of exercise potential. Your genetic makeup largely determines your max VO_2, so practically speaking, you cannot improve upon it. Of course, scientists already knew that the carbon dioxide/oxygen exchange could not be altered, so those two unchangeable factors led exercise physiologists to give little consideration to the possibility that a system of training could be built around breathing.

Though scientists understood that breathing itself is a mechanical action that is both involuntary and voluntary, they felt quite reluctant to suggest that athletes take control over such a vital physiological function. For example, you can overbreathe by taking lots of quick, short breaths. The result would be an unbalanced gas exchange and the release of too much carbon dioxide, and you would hyperventilate. (An aside:

The rhythmic patterns you will learn in this book call for longer inhalations and shorter exhalations.) So yes, if you mismanage your control of breathing, you could hyperventilate and become dizzy.

But the human body is a wonderful thing. It has remarkable systems in place to prevent serious harm. Every system in the body depends on oxygen, of course, including your life-sustaining cardiovascular, respiratory, and central nervous systems, which take first priority in the demand for oxygen. If, for example, during a run, your heart or your respiratory muscles were not getting enough blood, your brain would signal for vasoconstriction—tightening—of the arteries that feed your running muscles. Vasoconstriction of these arteries lessens bloodflow to these working muscles, allowing a greater volume of blood to reach the vital organs and muscles that are in need. When you run in extreme heat and humidity, constriction of the blood vessels to working muscles allows more bloodflow to the skin to facilitate cooling. The signal for these physiological actions comes from the brain and is automatic.

Muscle fatigue itself is a protective physiological response. Working muscle actually tires at about 65 percent of its full physiological capacity. Though muscle and brain together determine fatigue, world-renowned sports scientist Tim Noakes and his colleagues at the University of Cape Town identified what they called the Central Governor Model of Exercise Regulation, which posits that the central nervous system is at the forefront of slowing or stopping exercise long before complete physiological failure. The reason: to prevent harm.

So you see, even though you can control your breathing, your central nervous system has ultimate power. It monitors what's happening in your body and will usurp your control as necessary to protect your health. Managing breathing and oxygen during running can become a smooth and exhilarating dance between automatic and voluntary control of respiration once you learn the steps.

The Feel of Breathing

Breathing is so very conspicuous. We feel it. We see it (albeit indirectly). Sometimes we can even hear it. We don't notice the megawatts of nerve impulses zipping through our bodies to and from our central nervous system or the coursing of hormones carrying their messages. We are only barely aware of our beating heart—when we are at rest, anyway. But the breath—it is quite palpable.

TRY THIS: While sitting quietly at rest, focus on your breathing. Notice the air flowing in and out of your nostrils. Your abdomen and chest rise and fall. You can even count your breaths. Go ahead, count them, up to 10. Now focus on your heartbeat. Can you feel your heart beating in your chest? (Let's hope not.) Without putting your fingers to your pulse, can you count your heartbeats?

Not only can we control our breathing, but we can feel it and feel how it responds to work, and these qualities recommend breathing as an immediate physical gauge of our running effort. We can learn to measure the effort of running against the effort of breathing, making it an excellent training tool to help us quickly and smoothly make the needed adjustments for our best running performance.

Rhythmic Runner:
Craig Souders

RUNNER PROFILE: competitive runner; ran cross-country and track in college; PRs include 16:20 for 5-K, 34:20 for 10-K, 1:16:50 for the half, and 2:52 for the marathon

AGE: 36

OCCUPATION: physical therapist

> "Running is an aerobic sport, and breathing is the only way to monitor yourself in the moment."

Watches, heart rate monitors, Garmins . . . Craig Souders and Budd Coates agree that despite the advanced technology available to help with pacing, runners still go out too fast. "The Garmin says you are running fine . . . you are where you should be in the pack, but if you're not running within yourself, it doesn't matter," says Souders, who eagerly took to rhythmic breathing.

A competitive runner at every distance, Souders's current favorite is the 10-K. "I love the blend of speed and endurance that the 10-K requires," he says. "And at 36, I feel that my window for racing a good 10-K is closing."

Rhythmic breathing helps Soud-ers control his pace in training and racing, which, he says, makes both easier and more fun. "You really *do* feel like you're running on air," he enthuses.

"It's the only way to self-monitor," adds Souders. "Running is an aerobic sport, and breathing is the only way to monitor yourself in the moment." That ability to immediately connect with effort and pace have helped Souders become a better runner. "Even though my times are not as fast as when I was younger, I probably didn't race as well or as close to my potential [back then]," he says. "I feel like I am running proportionately better [now]." And on his way to a great 10-K.

CHAPTER 4

RHYTHMIC BREATHING

"To fine-tune your running, you've got to 'tune in.' You must feel your running. By learning to fit your breathing into your footsteps, you can increase your awareness while on the run." —Ian Jackson, athlete, coach, author

I n my early days as a runner, I, like most, didn't give any thought to my breathing as I ran. But when injury after injury sidelined me during my years at Springfield College, I went digging into the research to see if I could find a solution. My interest in breathing was sparked by references to running and breathing by Bill Bowerman (famed University of Oregon coach and co-founder of Nike) and author Ian Jackson. Both believed that breathing should be steady and rhythmic and coincide with footstrikes. Much the same as Thomas S. Miller, PhD and author of *Programmed to Run*, I found that serious running required longer inhalations than exhalations. Years later, I discovered that the greatest impact stress of running occurs when the foot strikes the ground at the beginning of exhalation and also that core stability is at its lowest during exhalation. I put these two precepts together with my knowledge of breathing and respiration to develop rhythmic breathing patterns that would help me avoid injury and train optimally for my best performance. It worked. I've taught this method to the many runners I've coached and advised over the years, and they've found that it has worked for them, too.

TRY THIS: To determine whether or not you breathe from your belly (diaphragm), lie on your back and place your hands on your belly. If your hands move up and down, you are using your diaphragm. If your hands remain still, you will most likely notice that your chest is moving up and down, which means you are depending too much on your intercostals—the small muscles that raise and lower your upper rib cage.

How to Breathe (Yes, Really)

Before learning the rhythmic patterns that will take your running to a new level, you must first become a belly breather. When you inhale, your diaphragm contracts and moves downward, while muscles in your chest contract to expand your rib cage. These actions increase the volume in your chest cavity and draw air into your lungs. Working your diaphragm to its fullest potential allows your lungs to expand to their greatest volume and fill with the largest amount of air. The more air you inhale, the more oxygen is available to be transferred through your circulatory system to your working muscles. Many people underuse their diaphragm, relying too much on their chest muscles and therefore taking in less oxygen, which is so important to energy production. The other downside of breathing from your chest is that these muscles (the intercostals) are smaller and will fatigue more quickly than your diaphragm will. Are you a belly breather or a chest breather?

If you are already a natural belly breather, terrific—you can move on to learn the rhythmic breathing patterns that will make you a better runner. If you breathe primarily with your chest muscles, however, you'll want to first train yourself to breathe with your diaphragm. Here's how:

- Lie down on your back.

- Keep your upper chest and shoulders still.

- Focus on raising your belly as you inhale.

- Lower your belly as you exhale.

- Inhale and exhale through both your nose and mouth.

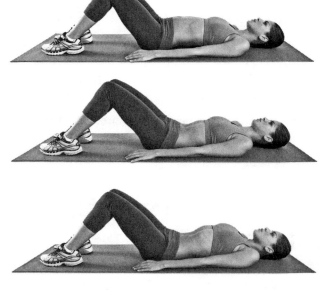

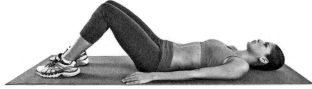

Belly breathing vs. chest breathing.

Practice belly breathing both lying down and sitting or standing, since you should be breathing diaphragmatically at all times—whether you're running, sleeping, eating, or reading a book.

How to Fit Breathing to Your Footstrikes

We've seen that the greatest impact force of running occurs when your foot strikes the ground at the point of exhale, and that your body is least stable during exhalation. And I've promised that by controlling your breathing, using rhythmic breathing, you can distribute that force evenly across your body and prevent injury. Here's how. Rhythmic breathing creates a relationship between your breathing cycle (inhale/exhale) and your stride cadence (footstrikes). And the singular point of all rhythmic breathing patterns that I will introduce to you in this book is this: Exhale on alternate footstrikes as you run. You never want to continuously exhale on the same foot. Many elite runners develop a 2:2 pattern of breathing. They inhale for two footstrikes and exhale for two footstrikes.

Every even-numbered breathing pattern, whether it's a 4-count (2:2) or 6-count (3:3), will have the same result. Breathing patterns based on odd numbers will shift the point of exhale alternately from left to right or right to left, from one side of the body to the other.

Let's start with a 5-count or 3:2 pattern of rhythmic breathing, which

The Longer Inhale

The rhythmic breathing patterns I recommend call for a longer inhale than exhale. You will either inhale for three steps and exhale for two or inhale two and exhale one. Why the longer inhale? Your diaphragm and other breathing muscles contract during inhalation, which brings stability to your core. These same muscles relax during exhalation, decreasing stability. With the goal of injury prevention in mind, it's best to hit the ground more often when your body is at its most stable—during inhalation.

will apply to most of your running. Inhale for three steps and exhale for two. Practice first on the floor:

1. Lie on your back with your knees bent and feet flat on the floor.

2. Place your hands on your belly and make sure that you are belly breathing.

3. Breathe through your nose and your mouth.

4. Inhale to the count of 3 and exhale to the count of 2. You might count it this way: "in-2-3," "out-2," "in-2-3," "out-2," and so forth.

5. Concentrate on a continuous breath as you inhale over the 3 counts and a continuous breath as you exhale.

6. Once you become comfortable with the inhale/exhale pattern, add foot taps to mimic walking steps.

When you feel confident that you have the 3:2 pattern down, take it for a walk. Inhale for three steps, exhale for two, inhale for three steps, exhale for two. You'll notice that this controlled pattern of breathing pushes the beginning of the exhale alternately from one foot to the other. Finally, of course, try out your rhythmic breathing on a run—inhaling for three footstrikes and exhaling for two, inhaling for three footstrikes and exhaling for two, and on and on. Here are a few key points to keep in mind:

• Inhale and exhale smoothly and continuously through both your nose and mouth.

• If it seems difficult to inhale over the full three strides, either inhale more gradually or pick up your pace.

• Do not listen to music while learning to breathe rhythmically. The beats of the music will confuse the heck out of you.

This pattern of rhythmic breathing will come easier to some than to others. Individuals with a singing or swimming background pick it up quickly. But trust me, it will eventually become second nature to anyone who chooses to use it. You won't have to think about it at all. You'll be able to hold a conversation while on a run, and rhythmic breathing will simply flow along with your running.

The Need to Breathe Faster

You will find that the 3:2 breathing pattern works well when you are running at an easy to moderate effort, which should make up the majority of your running. On an easy run, your breathing will be slower and more shallow than when you are running a little faster, a little harder—then you will breathe more deeply but still within the 3:2 breathing pattern. Let's say, however, you are out for a comfortable 5-miler and about midway you come upon a hill. Because your muscles are working harder, they need more oxygen. Your brain also signals to your respiratory system that you need to breathe faster and deeper.

You reach a point running up the hill when you can no longer comfortably inhale for three steps and exhale for two. It's time to then switch to a 3-count, or 2:1, rhythmic breathing pattern: inhale for two steps, exhale one, inhale two steps, exhale one. You're breathing faster, taking more breaths per minute, and this odd-numbered breathing pattern will continue to alternate the exhale from left foot to right, dispersing the impact stress of running equally across both sides of your body. Once you've crested the hill and are running down the other side, you might continue in this 2:1 pattern until your effort and breathing have recovered and you slip back into your 3:2 cadence.

TRY THIS: Get up and walk across the room. Inhale for two steps and exhale for two steps. You will see that the beginning of the exhale—the moment of peak impact stress—always occurs on the same foot.

When you begin breathing rhythmically, it's a good idea to consciously monitor your breathing patterns, although it's not necessary to do so throughout your entire run. Focus on your breathing when you start out, evaluate your breathing as your effort changes—such as when you climb a hill—and then simply check in at random intervals to make sure that you haven't fallen into a 2:2 pattern. Over time, the 3:2 and 2:1 rhythmic patterns will become automatic.

Not surprisingly, the 2:1 breathing pattern also comes into play during speed training and racing. I originally began to use rhythmic breathing as a way to run injury-free. When I realized it was working with easy and moderate runs, I was afraid to break away from it during hard training workouts, and through trial and error I learned to alter my breathing between the 5- and 3-count patterns. I followed a 5-count rhythmic breathing pattern during an easy run or a long run and a 3-count rhythm for interval training and racing. Rhythmic breathing allowed me to complete my last year of competitive college running with moderate success, earning my one and only varsity letter in cross-country and successfully finishing my first marathon.

How to Gauge Your Effort (Feel Your Running)

Any runner who wants to take it to the next level and compete—whether their goal is the local 5-K or to qualify for the Boston Marathon—must vary the distance, terrain, and pace of his or her daily runs. The ability to properly gauge and control the effort of each of those workouts is the runner's most valuable training tool. Yes, as we discussed earlier, you can use a heart rate monitor to measure the effort of your workouts. But remember, the heart monitor is an intermediary, the middleman, so to speak, in the effort-control equation of running.

Measuring effort through rhythmic breathing puts you directly in touch with your body, provides immediate feedback, and gives you complete control over your effort and pace. You can respond more quickly to your body's need for oxygen, which will make your effort smoother and more efficient, and make running more comfortable.

Smooth and efficient running equals faster running at any given level of effort.

It's analogous to driving a car with an automatic transmission versus driving a car that employs a manual transmission. The automatic transmission—like the heart monitor—senses the effort of the engine for you and then will shift gears as needed. With manual transmission, you must tune in to your car—listen to the engine and feel its effort—then you shift into the appropriate gear. With practice and experience at gauging/feeling the effort, you will have greater control. Consider this: Race cars are equipped with manual transmission, not automatic. And yes, race cars burn a lot of fuel, but in general, a manual transmission saves on gas. The runner who shifts running gears manually also enjoys greater efficiency.

The Rhythmic Breathing Effort Key

As we've seen, the 5-count (3:2) rhythmic breathing pattern suits slow to moderate running. You'll shift to the 3-count (2:1) pattern for faster running and racing. Of course, a complete training program requires more than two speeds. An optimal mix of workouts includes slow, moderate, and fast running, hills, and flat terrain. After developing the 5- and 3-count running patterns, I spent a few years combining those patterns with different types of training and eventually I created the Rhythmic Breathing Effort Scale that you'll find on page 36. For the framework of this scale, I turned to the Borg Rating of Perceived Exertion Scale, developed by Gunnar Borg, PhD. The Borg Scale ranks effort from 0 to 20 based on one's evaluation of breathlessness and fatigue during exercise, with 0 representing no activity and 20 representing maximum effort. Eventually, the scale was condensed to a simpler 10-digit ranking called the Borg CR10 Scale.

Borg Rating of Perceived Exertion Scale

BORG 0-20	CR10	EFFORT
0-8	0-0.5	total rest to light task while standing
9-10	1-2	very light work
11-12	3	light work
13-14	4	somewhat hard
15-16	5-6	hard
17-18	7-8	very hard
19-20	9-10	maximum, all-out work

Since I needed to define a range of efforts within the easier 5-count breathing pattern and within the harder 3-count pattern, I saw that I could use the Borg Scale to further divide these two broad efforts. And I could create one scale—one training tool—that would inform the runner as to what breathing pattern to use and at what effort.

I developed three levels of effort within the 5-count (3:2) breathing pattern and three levels within the 3-count (2:1) pattern. Then I added a seventh level of effort above and beyond the 2:1 pattern, which represents the all-out effort required of sprint workouts, race surges, and race finishes. I assigned each level a number that indicates the breathing pattern (5 or 3) and effort (1, 2, or 3). So, for example, 51 means that you run in the 5-count breathing pattern at the easiest effort, 52 is a little harder, and 53, harder still. Next comes 31, which is the point at which you need to switch to the 3-count pattern of breathing, followed by 32, then 33. Here's the rhythmic breathing scale in its entirety:

Rhythmic Breathing Effort (RBE) Scale

The first number of the RBE represents the breathing pattern; the second number represents the effort level within that pattern.

RBE	EFFORT	BORG SCALE
51	easy running, slow, little effort	9–10
52	moderate effort, slightly tiring, middle to long distance	11–12
53	fast aerobic run, close to over the edge	13–14
31	race pace (effort) for half and full marathon	15–16
32	race pace (effort) for 5-K to 10-K	17–18
33	race pace (effort) for 1 mile and intervals	19
2:1:1:1	short intervals, surges, hills, and race finishes	20

And yes, it includes one more breathing pattern for those moments when you run all out. This breathing pattern uses the 3-count pattern followed by a one-step inhale and a one-step exhale. So you will breathe in for two steps, exhale one step, inhale one step, exhale one step. And you will repeat the pattern for the short duration of your sprint or surge.

The Rhythmic Breathing Effort Scale (RBE) works for runners of all abilities—whether you run a 5-K in 36 minutes or 13, a half-marathon in 2 hours or 1, a marathon in 5 hours or 2½—because rhythmic breathing uses effort to guide workouts. You and elite runners such as Ryan Hall and Kara Goucher will all run your easy runs at an RBE of 51. It's not pace that counts, but effort. Focusing on how fast you run a particular workout pushes you to work your body harder than what might be appropriate. It pushes you to overtrain, which slows recovery and can even prevent full recovery from workouts, and this simply snowballs into poor-quality workouts and poor performance. Plus, it's not fun.

Let's look at a hypothetical but very realistic example. You're really busy at work; your kids' baseball games, dance recital, and school play have all converged on the next 2 weeks; you haven't been sleeping well. You head out the door for a 5-miler. You get to the 1-mile point and check your watch—Ugh!—You are so slow today. But you're training for a half-marathon and you think you should be running faster, so you pick up the pace even though it's uncomfortable. You finish your run feeling that it's been an unsatisfying struggle. Rather than take a more relaxed approach to your training, you continue to push over the next few weeks. Race day arrives. You struggle through to a disappointing finish.

The beauty of rhythmic breathing is that it teaches you to run within yourself. You won't overtrain on any given day. You won't fight with your body to do more than it should. You listen to your body, and you run at the effort prescribed according to your ability on that day. And when it comes time to race, you will be perfectly trained to achieve your best performance.

Learning Your Rhythmic Breathing Effort

It is easy enough to find that point when you need to switch from the 5-count (3:2) breathing pattern to the 3-count (2:1) pattern. The 5-count pattern simply becomes too uncomfortable to maintain and you must breathe faster. But how will you know when you are running at 52 or at 53? Or 32 or 33? The answer is that you will *feel* it. It comes with practice, with trial and error. And it all starts with focus. You must pay attention to how you feel, the effort of your breathing, as you run.

On your next run, do some "breath play," as Ian Jackson would say. Start out in a 5-count breathing pattern at a very easy effort—your warmup. This is a comfortable pace that you could maintain for a long run without fatigue, a pace at which you could converse easily with a running partner. This is a rhythmic breathing effort (RBE) of 51. How does it feel? Notice the depth and rate of your breathing.

After 10 minutes, pick up your pace just a bit to an effort that requires you to breathe noticeably deeper while you continue to run within the 5-count breathing pattern—a pace that is comfortably fast. You should still be able to talk with your running buddy, but you'll be glad for those periods in the conversation when you get to listen to your friend talking. You are now at a rhythmic breathing effort of 52. Run at this pace for a

Sex Differences

Though I've taught the rhythmic breathing program the same way to women as I have to men, women may have a slightly different experience because of differences in respiratory mechanics. Women generally have a smaller lung volume than men (for details, see J.A. Guenette's work listed in the bibliography). This means that women may need to convert from a 5-count pattern to a 3-count pattern or from a 3-count pattern to a 2:1:1:1 pattern before a man would, and more often during a strenuous run or race.

For example, imagine you're a woman out for a moderate run over a course that includes a few hills. Late in the run, fatigue begins setting in, which means the pace feels harder, and then you start to climb a hill. You should keep this run at an RBE of 51, but halfway up the hill you find that your Rhythmic Breathing Effort moves quickly straight through 52 to 53, yet you aren't pushing the pace. What to do? Simply convert to a 3-count pattern, a 31, while running a comfortable pace until you crest the hill. Ease into the downhill and, as comfort allows, return to a 51 RBE.

What happened? The work required to conquer the hill demanded an increase in oxygen, but you can fill your lungs with only so much air, and the 5-count pattern wasn't allowing you enough breaths per minute to meet this need. Switching to the three-step pattern allowed you more breaths and oxygen per minute. Young athletes—male or female—who are still developing may have the same experience.

Guys, depending on the length or height of the hill, may experience the same issue. Keith Livingstone, author of *Healthy Intelligent Training*, points out that few courses are perfect for an aerobic run. Most will deliver a challenge or two along the way.

few minutes and tune in to your body, feel your breathing—your lungs expanding, your belly rising.

Now pick up your pace even further while holding the 5-step breathing pattern. At this point, you'll be breathing about as deeply as you can, which makes the effort uncomfortable. You may be able to spit out a few words before you are forced to concentrate on your breathing, and you will feel a need to breathe faster. You are now experiencing rhythmic breathing effort 53. And you'd rather not.

So let's convert to a 3-step breathing pattern—inhaling for two steps and exhaling for one. This allows you to breathe faster. Notice that the effort of breathing becomes comfortable again. You will be able to talk some, but you won't be carrying on a monologue. Running will feel comfortably fast again, as it did when you were at an RBE of 52; but you are now at an RBE of 31 and able to run faster than you could at 52. Again, spend a few minutes at this pace and effort, focusing on your breathing and on your body. By tuning in, you will become more familiar with how your body feels, and over time these levels of effort will come more naturally—you will be running with the rhythms of your body.

Now increase your pace, forcing deeper breathing. You are running at a serious level that does not allow you to talk, and breathing is deep but manageable. This is RBE 32. Up the pace again. The effort will feel similar to what you experienced when running at a rhythmic breathing effort of 53. You are breathing about as deeply as you can, but the difference is that you are also breathing about as fast as you can. And, of course, your pace is much quicker. You've now reached RBE 33 on the Rhythmic Breathing Effort Scale, and you can't hold this effort for too long.

At an RBE of 33, it might feel like you have no place else to go, but you do—RBE 2:1:1:1, which allows you to breathe faster. As you give this level a test run, you can choose to pick up the pace or not. Focus on your breathing pattern, because you're going to switch to the following: inhale for two steps, exhale for one, inhale for one, exhale for one; inhale for two steps, exhale for one, inhale for one, exhale for one; and so forth. You are taking in more breaths per minute, which will help you maintain, even increase slightly, the pace you were running at 33. This is the effort you will put forth for your kick at the end of a race. Or, as you'll see in the racing chapter, you can use this RBE to help you crest a steep hill during a race. The 2:1:1:1 rhythmic breathing effort is the sharpest beat of your body's running rhythms, where your quickest pace (or hardest effort) and fastest breaths meet.

Once you've tested the 2:1:1:1 RBE, slow down, ease up, and allow your breathing to return to a comfortable 51. This won't happen all at once. You may instead find yourself running easily but still needing to breathe at the faster rate of a 3-count pattern. Eventually, however, you

Five Training Zones

To help both athletes and individuals new to exercise understand and monitor the effort and intensity of their workouts, coaches and trainers commonly use the 5 Training Zone method for defining intensity, with zone 1 representing the easiest effort and zone 5 representing the hardest. These zones can be defined by percentage of lactate threshold, max VO_2, or maximum heart rate, but since we can easily measure heart rate, it is used most often. The Rhythmic Breathing Effort Scale correlates nicely with these five training zones (see table below). Rhythmic breathing efforts fall within intersecting circles of intensity: 53 and 31 can occur at the same pace, as can 33 and 2:1:1:1. The difference is the breathing pattern. If you are accustomed to using a heart rate monitor and the 5 Training Zone method to measure your exercise intensity, you can instead use rhythmic breathing for the same purpose and leave your heart rate monitor at home.

TRAINING ZONES	RHYTHMIC BREATHING EFFORT
Zone 1	RBE 51
Zone 2	RBE 52
Zone 3	RBE 53 and 31
Zone 4	RBE 32
Zone 5	RBE 33 and 2:1:1:1

will settle into a rhythmic breathing effort of 51 for your cooldown. Don't hesitate to play with these rhythmic breathing efforts during other runs. The more you use rhythmic breathing in training and racing, the easier and more automatic it becomes.

A few nuances to consider: When you run a pace that coincides with your easiest RBE of 51, you cannot force that pace to feel like a 52 or 53 unless you run for a long time. Fatigue increases your perceived exertion, and when you are tired the same level of work feels harder. But keeping the pace the same, you can change your RBE from a 51 to a 31 simply by switching from a 5-count pattern to a 3-count pattern—slower breathing to faster breathing. The point is, as we discussed in Chapter 3, you have some control over your breathing. You likely will never choose to breathe faster at your easiest pace, but at harder paces and efforts, changing your breathing rate will allow you to maintain your pace because the effort will feel more comfortable. Know, too, that the Rhythmic Breathing Effort Scale is a guide to help you discover your own levels of effort and pace. As you use rhythmic breathing in your training and racing and tune in to your breathing efforts and paces, you will learn to run from within, in complete harmony with your body. You will discover the natural rhythms of your running, which will lead you to improved performances but also to experience the pure joy of running.

Rhythmic Runner:
Richard Ryan

RUNNER PROFILE: competitive runner—high school, college, postcollege; in 2010, he finished 13th in Philadelphia's 10-mile Broad Street Run in 52:50

AGE: 26

OCCUPATION: event marketing, Brooks shoe company

> "It helps you to understand where your fitness is and what you are capable of doing."

Rich Ryan has never bought in to the thinking that everything about how to train and race for optimal performance is already known. He's always looking to discover something new, to try something different. So when he met Budd Coates at the Christmas City Classic in Bethlehem, Pennsylvania, in December 2011 and the conversation turned to rhythmic breathing, Ryan's interest was piqued. "I knew about Budd's accomplishments. He has a lot of credibility," says Ryan, who eagerly dug into the material Coates sent him about rhythmic breathing.

"I bought in right away," he adds. "It took me a couple of runs to get the patterns down. And I messed around with it a little— I tried inhaling for four steps and exhaling for three, which was a little dizzying," he says with a chuckle, "so I scaled back to the 5-count [recommended] pattern."

Rhythmic breathing has allowed Ryan to tune in to his body and run according to effort. "It's self-regulating. Before, my training was based on time and watches," he explains. "Now I don't check my splits during a workout. Rhythmic breathing quantifies effort, allowing you to run by effort.

"It helps you to understand where your fitness is and what you are capable of doing," he adds. "And you develop an excellent sense of pace."

All of these attributes have propelled Ryan to great performances. In 2011, having begun to use rhythmic breathing in the spring, he ran an 8-K in 25 minutes flat and continued to improve. "My best streak of running started in November 2011," says Ryan. And as of this writing, that streak was still going strong.

CHAPTER 5

BEGINNING RUNNING

"The journey of a thousand miles begins beneath one's feet."—Lao Tzu, Chinese philosopher

Most of us have started something—a hobby, a home project, a diet, a fitness routine—only to abandon it after a few months, maybe even a few weeks. Most often, it's not because of a lack of willpower but instead lack of know-how, lack of a clear goal with clear objectives, and lack of a reasonable plan for achieving that goal. Yes, a journey of a thousand miles begins beneath your feet. And filled with excitement for your new venture, you press forward, logging as many steps as you can, day after day, toward your lofty goal until you become fatigued, sore, bored, injured, or all of the above. And then you quit.

I have taught beginning running for more than 30 years, and over and over I see this beginner's exuberance coupled with a lack of understanding about how to progress smartly. I see new runners make two key mistakes when they start a running program. First, they run too fast. Though most will say, "I'm too old" or "I'm too overweight" or "I'm too slow to run fast," they all run faster than they should. The effort is difficult and uncomfortable, and they cannot run very far at all.

If you are new to running, focus not on pace but on effort—a calm, controlled, relaxed effort. The "talk test" is the well-known gauge of effort recommended for beginners and a perfect gauge of rhythmic breathing. You should be able to comfortably carry on a conversation while you run. As we discussed in Chapter 4, that effort is a 51 on the Rhythmic Breathing Effort Scale. If you find that you can only manage a word or two of conversation before gasping for a breath, you are running a bit too fast—a rhythmic breathing effort (RBE) of 52 or 53. And you should slow down.

The second mistake many new runners make is that they run too far. Any distance is a journey into the unknown, and so the beginning runner heads down the street or trail and keeps running until he or she can't go any farther. Running too fast and too far makes one's breathing labored and uncomfortable. Do that day after day and it's not surprising that you might give up running altogether. Worse yet, you could become injured and be forced to stop. Running at a comfortable pace for a comfortable period of time allows your body to adapt and grow stronger.

The beginning running program I've developed mixes minutes of running with minutes of walking for a total of 30 minutes—there's no need to be concerned about mileage. Alternating minutes of walking with minutes of running follows the same principle of interval training that an elite runner would use to train his or her body to run stronger and faster. You perform a hard effort (the running minutes) with recovery (the walking minutes) and, over time, your body adapts to this effort and gets stronger. The difference for the beginner versus the elite runner is only in the pace at a given effort.

But even the elite runner can benefit from walking. The great Czech runner Emil Zatopek, who won gold in the 5000 meters, 10,000 meters, and marathon at the 1952 Olympics in Helsinki—setting Olympic records in all three events—would take long breaks from running, followed by long sessions over wooded trails with endless combinations of walking and easy running intervals.

Before starting the beginning running program, you must first be able to walk continuously for 30 minutes at least three times a week. Start with a 15-minute walk three times a week; the next week, bump up the walk to 20 minutes; and the following week, move up to 25 minutes of walking. Finally, increase your walks to 30-minutes on 3 days with a day of rest between. As you walk, remember to focus on the 5-count rhythmic breathing pattern: Inhale for three footsteps and exhale for two. You can walk as briskly as you like, as long as you can maintain the 5-count (3:2) breathing pattern.

Learning to Exhale

A runner once came to me after a few failed attempts at beginning a running program on her own. She had been making the common new-runner mistake of running too fast, so I taught her rhythmic breathing and got her started on week one. After just a few workouts she complained that she was having trouble inhaling as she ran, because every time she tried to do so, she still had air in her lungs. I hadn't heard this one before and, quite honestly, it had me a bit perplexed. But I gave it some thought and came to understand what was happening.

When we are at rest, we exhale without any effort. As we begin to exercise, we inhale deeper and have to push air out as we exhale. Our expiratory muscles (the muscles used during exhalation) need to contract more forcefully to force air out more quickly. This runner's inability to do this was a cognitive disconnect with her breathing. I taught her how to use her expiratory muscles properly, and when she applied this skill while running it became second nature. She sailed through the beginning running program.

WARMING UP, COOLING DOWN

Before you begin your walk or run, a gentle transition from being at rest to becoming active—called a warmup—prepares your body for the increased work and movement of running. Likewise, a stretching cooldown provides a gentle transition from the hard work of running to a state of rest. It's like driving—smooth acceleration and braking are healthier for your car than putting the pedal to the metal or slamming on the brakes.

Warmup

The following short series of exercises will get your blood moving a little faster and loosen up muscles and joints. Perform them in the order shown.

Hip Circles

With feet shoulder-width apart, circle your hips as if you are hula-hooping. Perform 8 rotations, then circle your hips in the opposite direction.

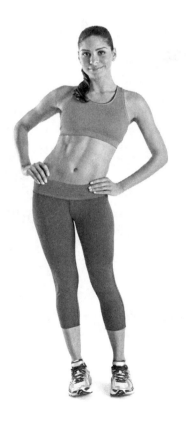
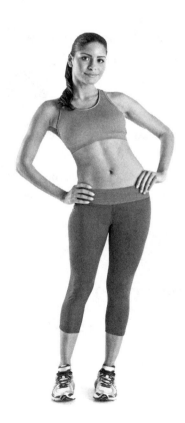

Body Lean

With feet slightly more than shoulder-width apart and hands behind your head, lean to the left and then to the right. Repeat 7 times.

Dance Kicks

Stand with your right side near a wall, tree, pole, or other firm surface and place your right hand on that surface for support. Swing your left leg forward, backward, and then out to the side. Complete this sequence 7 times and repeat on the opposite side of your body.

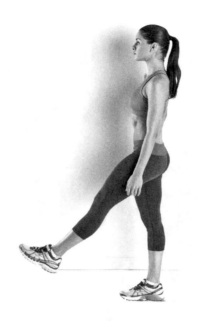

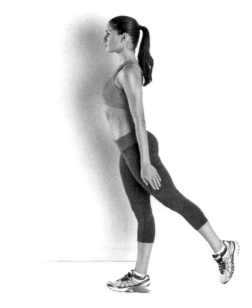

Calf Raise

Stand with your right side near a wall, tree, pole, or other firm surface and place your right hand on that surface for support. Lift your left foot entirely off the ground and bring the heel of your right foot up and off the ground, then gently lower. Repeat 7 times and then switch sides.

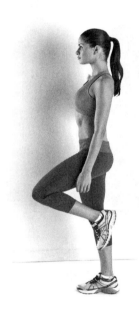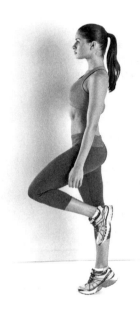

Cooldown

A stretching cooldown after every run prevents loss of flexibility in your muscles and helps you stay injury-free. On the following pages are five essential stretches for new runners.

Lower Back and Hamstring Stretch

Stand with feet shoulder-width apart and hands clasped behind your back. Keep your legs straight and lean forward as far as you can while raising your hands as high as you can. Hold for 8–20 seconds. From this position, release your hands and reach down and grasp your lower legs. Pull slightly to increase the stretch and hold for another 8–20 seconds. Bend your knees, release your hands, and slowly straighten up.

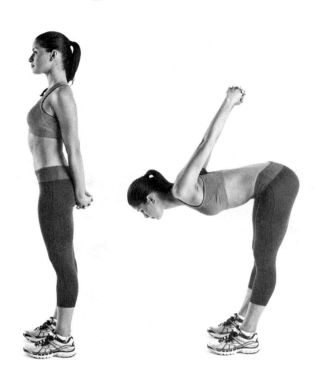

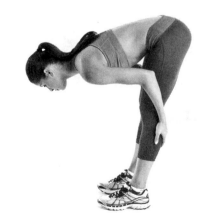

Straight-Leg Calf Stretch

Stand a little more than an arm's length away from a wall, tree, or other firm surface. Extend your arms forward at shoulder height and lean toward the wall, placing your palms against it. Bring your right foot forward while keeping your left foot flat on the ground and your left knee straight. Move your hips toward the wall and bend your arms, if needed, to feel the stretch in your calf. Hold for 8–20 seconds and repeat on the opposite side.

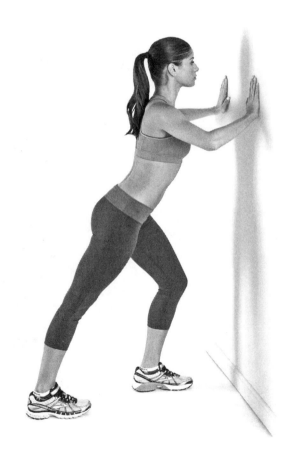

Bent–Leg Calf Stretch

Repeat the straight-leg calf stretch on page 53, but bend the back of your knee.

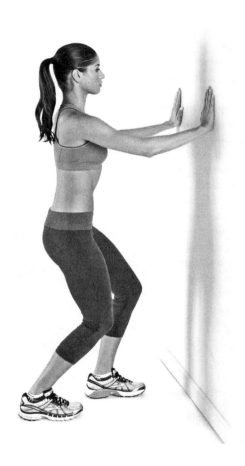

Quad/Hamstring Stretch

Stand with your feet shoulder-width apart and a little more than an arm's length away from a wall, tree, or other firm surface. Extend your arms forward at shoulder height and lean toward the wall, placing your palms against it. Reach back with your right hand and grasp your right ankle behind you. Pull your ankle as high as possible while leaning forward from your hip (keep your left leg straight). Hold for 8–20 seconds, then repeat on the opposite side.

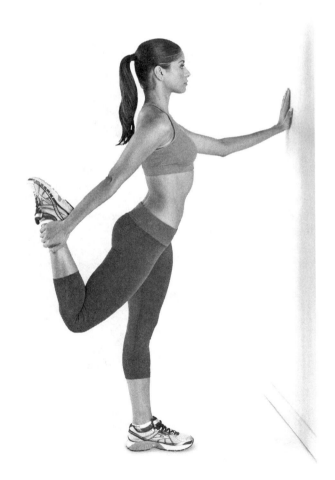

Hip/Iliotibial Band Stretch

Stand with your feet together and your right side facing a wall, tree, or other firm surface about an arm's length away. Lean toward the wall, extending your right arm straight out to the wall for support. Keeping your legs and arm straight, push your hips toward the wall, rotating the left hip slightly forward, and hold for 8–20 seconds. Repeat on the opposite side.

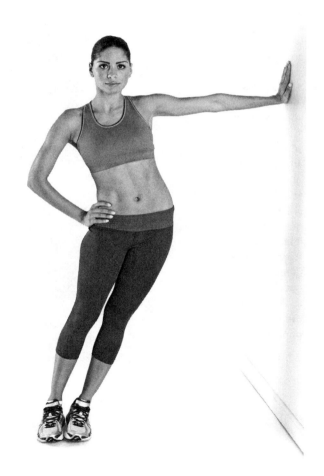

Running Form

If I've been asked once, I've been asked a million times about proper running form.

Running form is a lot like a signature—it's yours, and you can be identified by it. Recently, while I was finishing up a run, a longtime friend hollered out, "I knew that form as soon as I pulled into the parking lot." Runners and coaches can pick out other runners from great distances by spotting their signature form, and running form can vary greatly among very successful athletes. Perhaps this is why it gets little attention.

When I was a freshman at Springfield College I competed at the 1976 Boston College Relays. I remember watching a high school boy competing in the open 10-K against some of the best runners from the Greater Boston Track Club (Bill Rodgers was among them). This high schooler ran bent over so far from his waist that it appeared as if he was attempting to tie his shoes. That kid was Alberto Salazar, and he fared quite well that night. He went on to become an international force in the marathon with what was referred to as a marathon shuffle, and he competed at the international level on the indoor and outdoor track and shorter road race distances. If he could be successful with his obvious form flaws, why should we be concerned? He wasn't the exception, either. Many world record holders have had questionable form, including Jim Ryun and Haile Gebrselassie.

Running Buddies

Studies show that when you have a partner to exercise with, you are more likely to stick with your program. The same goes for running. Perhaps enlist a friend to take up running, too. You will help make each other accountable to the schedule, and when you're running together, you can easily use the talk test to make sure you stay at a comfortable level of effort. Just be careful not to get so caught up in conversation that you forget to check in on your rhythmic breathing every now and then. As a beginner, you'll want to make sure you are maintaining the 5-count (3:2) pattern and haven't slipped into a 2:2 pattern.

Today, Salazar is coach to a double gold medalist from the London Olympics, Mo Farah; a silver medalist in the 10,000 meters, American Galen Rupp; and a host of other world-class distance runners. Salazar pays as much attention to his athletes' form as he does their training and diet. He believes that form breaks can add seconds to a runner's time—and seconds can be the difference between winning and watching.

For some of us, bad form and/or form breaks that occur when we're fatigued may be the cause of recurring injury. "If you're not in the right form, and if you can't hold that form, you're going to stay in that injury cycle," says musculoskeletal therapist Phil Wharton.

According to Salazar and Wharton, ignoring form may come at a price to performance and health. But not everyone agrees that attention to running form has much value. "For most people, I don't know if focusing on form is of great benefit," says Pete Rea, elite athlete coach and coordinator at the ZAP Fitness Team USA Training Center. "It appeals to our need for the perfect pill or magic bullet, to figure out the secret. When, really, there is no secret."

There's also much debate over what defines good form. Of late, chi running, which emphasizes the core; barefoot running, which forces a forefoot strike; and the pose method, which is based on an S-like position of the body, have received the most attention as the best way to prevent injury. While many everyday runners have adopted these methods, elite and world-class runners have not, for the most part, found them of value.

What *can* we agree on? Following are guidelines that apply to all runners of all abilities.

- Your body should have a slight forward lean as you run, such that a straight line could be drawn from your heel just before takeoff through your hips, core, and head.

- Though the jury is still out on where your foot should first hit the ground (I recommend a midfoot strike), at footstrike your knee should be slightly bent and your foot should be under, not in front of, your body.

- Your elbows should be bent at 90 degrees or less and should swing from behind your body to your ribs but not pass in front of your body.

- Your hands should be relaxed but not flopping. Some like to imagine holding a potato chip; I like holding my thumb inside a loose fist. They should swing toward a point in front of your body but not cross your body.

- Your head should be upright (keep in mind that line from your heel), with eyes focused ahead, not on the ground immediately in front of you.

These guidelines should be simple to follow, but if you find any of them difficult to master, seek a running coach who understands biomechanics to assist you. Small changes in form will require very little adaptation from your joints and muscles, but significant changes can cause injuries if you do not take the time to allow your joints and muscles to adapt. Back off on mileage and quality workouts until your body feels comfortable in its new posture.

The Beginning Running Program

I hear plenty of people say they like the idea of becoming a runner but that running is difficult and just too much work—it's not fun. And I would bet that many of those individuals tried running, made the mistakes of running too fast and too long, and quit after a couple of weeks. The following 10-week program *eases* you into running. I promise that if you stick to the recommended workouts and use rhythmic breathing to keep your effort easy, these run/walk sessions will feel comfortable. To flip the well-worn axiom, it's a case of no pain resulting in tremendous gain. I have taught this program to a few thousand new runners, and, not to blow my own horn, I've had 100 percent success. Now that you can walk comfortably for 30 minutes, you are ready to run.

WORKOUT CHECKLIST

- Use a sports watch so you can time the walk and run segments.

- All of these workouts should be performed at an RBE of 51. Follow the 5-count breathing pattern (inhale for three steps, exhale for two) and maintain an easy effort (level 1) that allows you to talk easily as you walk and run.

- Walk for 2 to 3 minutes before the start of each workout to get comfortable with rhythmic breathing.

- Each of the workouts lasts 30 minutes.

- Cool down with stretching.

- Plan to do each 30-minute run/walk at least three times during the week—preferably with a day off between workouts—before moving up to the next week's workouts.

First Marathons

While I recommend that new runners not progress beyond 20 miles (about 200 minutes) per week during their first 6 to 12 months or race longer than a 10-K, I did break this rule myself back in 1987. To raise more funds in our United Way campaign at Rodale Inc., I was asked to coach 50 local businessmen and women to run the New York City Marathon. In return, each participant had to collect a minimum of $1,500 in donations for the United Way. Thirteen of those participants were experienced runners and simply needed to fine-tune their training. The other 37 had either never run a step or had not for quite some time. These 37 individuals completed my 10-week beginning running program and then moved into the Schedule A marathon training program you'll find starting on page 129. In the end, 36 of the 37 new runners, along with the 13 veterans, finished the marathon and raised more than $80,000 for the United Way. So, while I don't recommend that you run a marathon in your first year as a runner, be assured that it is possible. But your only goal should be to finish healthy.

Week1

WORKOUT: Run 2 minutes, walk 4 minutes (perform this sequence 5 times; total of 30 minutes)

Notes: Run only as fast as or just slightly faster than your brisk walk. If you feel as though you can't catch your breath, you're going too fast.

Slow to a walk, recover your breathing, and start over at a slower pace. Each 2-minute running interval should create a little tiredness but not exhaustion. After running for 2 minutes, the 4-minute walk that follows should be restful and allow you to recover and feel fresh for the next 2-minute run.

Week2

WORKOUT: Run 3 minutes, walk 3 minutes (perform this sequence 5 times)

Notes: Once you start to run, pay close attention to your breathing

pattern and adjust your running pace to keep your breathing under control. Remember, the amount of work you do will determine how fast and/or deep you need to breathe. When you slow your pace, your breathing will become more manageable.

Week3

WORKOUT: Run 5 minutes, walk 2½ minutes (perform this sequence 4 times)

Notes: As you progress to longer and longer running segments, it will become increasingly important to maintain your rhythmic breathing pattern, so continue to pay close attention. While the 2½-minute walk is all

the recovery you'll need between running segments, if you find it difficult to keep track, simply walk for 3 minutes between runs instead. You'll repeat this sequence three times for a total of 20 minutes of running and 10 to 12 minutes of walking. In just 3 weeks, you've doubled the amount of time you can run within the 30 minutes. Great job!

Week4

WORKOUT: Run 7 minutes, walk 3 minutes (perform this sequence 3 times)

Notes: One nice aspect of the longer running segments is that you don't repeat them as many times. Remember to breathe through both your mouth and nose to move as much oxygen into the body as possible and to release carbon dioxide.

Week5

WORKOUT: Run 8 minutes, walk 2 minutes (perform this sequence 3 times)

Notes: Along with the running segments getting longer, the walking segments are getting rather short, and you may be tempted to walk them at a brisk pace. The purpose of these walking breaks is to allow your muscles a chance to regroup so you can repeat the longer running segment with relative ease. If you walk too briskly, you will build up too much fatigue and may be forced to stop your workout early. Stay relaxed.

Week6

WORKOUT: Run 9 minutes, walk 2 minutes; repeat; then run 8 minutes

Notes: That's right—run 9 minutes, walk 2 minutes, run 9, walk 2, and finish with 8 minutes of running for a total of 30 minutes. Finish off this workout with 1 to 2 minutes of walking before your cooldown routine.

Week 7

WORKOUT: Run 9 minutes, walk 1 minute (perform this sequence 3 times)

Notes: Though this stage looks a lot like week 6, the 1-minute recovery walk makes a difference. You'll only be recovering for half as long as you did last week. Don't worry, though. If you use rhythmic breathing, you'll sail through.

Week 8

WORKOUT: Run 13 minutes, walk 2 minutes (perform this sequence twice)

Notes: The running segments have increased by 4 minutes in this stage, but your recovery walk is doubled to 2 minutes. That recovery, and the fact that you only do this sequence twice, makes this workout very doable. As these running segments get longer, it is very important that you make sure the pace is slow enough to allow you to keep your rhythmic breathing under control (inhale 3, exhale 2) and comfortable (you should be able to have a conversation). Also, with these longer running segments you're no doubt starting to cover some distance. If you run on a trail, bike path, or other straight course, you can now run one way for the first segment, continue the same direction during the walk, and then turn around and head for home for the second half of the workout.

Week 9

WORKOUT: Run 14 minutes, walk 1 minute (perform this sequence twice)

Notes: What a difference 1 minute makes! I've robbed a minute from your walk and given it to your run. Remember to walk slowly during that minute, allowing you to recover as much as possible.

Week10

WORKOUT: Run 30 minutes

Notes: Yes, you are ready to run the entire workout. First walk for 1 to 2 minutes to get into the rhythmic breathing pattern; then ease into the run. This is your first long run. Remember, it's not how fast you run; the goal is just to run for 30 continuous minutes. Now, I've heard countless times that it's just too big a jump, from 14 minutes to 30, but it's not. Trust me. You no longer need that minute walk you were taking last week, as long as you watch your effort. That said, I'm going to share a little rhythmic breathing trick with you. If you start to feel a bit over-fatigued as you near the 20-minute mark, or anytime thereafter, convert your breathing pattern to two breaths in and one breath out. This will allow you to get nearly twice as many full breaths of air per minute, increasing the oxygen flow to your working muscles and, in turn, turbo-boosting your performance. Congratulations, you did it! You're now a runner.

28 Reasons to Run

1. Fast, efficient way to cardiovascular fitness
2. Excellent way to lose/manage weight
3. Reduces blood triglycerides (fat)
4. Lowers total cholesterol
5. Raises HDL (good cholesterol)
6. Prevents stiffening of arteries that comes with age
7. Lowers blood pressure
8. Reduces risk of stroke
9. Reduces risk of breast cancer
10. Enhances immune system
11. Helps prevent and manage diabetes
12. Keeps intestinal tract functioning well
13. May reduce symptoms of asthma
14. May ease PMS
15. Improves health during pregnancy
16. May ease symptoms of menopause
17. Preserves bone and muscle mass
18. Improves flexibility and range of motion in joints
19. Stimulates development of neurons in brain
20. Helps lift depression
21. Boosts energy
22. Relieves stress
23. Stimulates creativity
24. Helps you feel happy
25. Boosts confidence through accomplishment
26. Provides opportunity to compete
27. Can run for a lifetime
28. It's fun!

Running On

So you can run for 30 minutes. Now what? It's time to decide what kind of runner you want to be. Think about your goals. Is running your choice for maintaining good health? Running can help you manage your weight, cholesterol, and blood pressure. It can help lift depression and give you a new outlook on life. Or perhaps you want to race—the local 5-K or Thanksgiving Turkey Trot. Maybe you dream of completing a marathon one day. And, of course, your running goals can and may evolve as you continue to run.

If your reason for becoming a runner is to improve or maintain your overall fitness and health, a schedule that gets you out the door 3 to 5 days a week will meet your needs. The 14-day cycle on page 85 shows you how to plan your runs and rest days for optimal performance, and by varying the time (distance) you run, you'll stay healthy as your fitness improves. How much running you do depends on your specific health goals and what fits comfortably into your lifestyle.

Want to enter an upcoming 5-K? Go ahead. Once you've completed the beginning running program, you are ready. Your first 5-K might take you a little longer than 30 minutes. It might take you a little less. But if you monitor your effort through your breathing and keep it comfortable, I guarantee you can run from the start right on through the finish line. But even if you need to take a short walking break at the water stop, who cares? When you're ready, ease back into a comfortable running effort and head for the finish.

If you have a few weeks before your first race, advance to Schedule A on page 98. Continue to work up from one schedule to the next until the long run in the cycle is equal to or longer (50 percent longer is ideal, except for the marathon) than your goal race distance. A word of caution: Do not do too much too soon. The first priority of this book is to teach you to run in tune with your body and to make that connection through breathing. As you progress through the schedules provided in

Treadmill Running

You'll find times when running on a treadmill is an excellent, if not necessary, alternative to running outdoors. Perhaps the weather is extraordinarily cold, rainy, or hot and humid. Maybe you're on a business trip or vacationing in an unfamiliar city. My reason for buying a treadmill was that my children were young and I couldn't leave the house.

You can do any of your scheduled workouts on the treadmill. I've programmed all of my outdoor courses on my 23-year-old Precor: my 5-mile morning run, 13-mile parks loop, and yes, even my 22-mile Waiatarua Circuit hill loop. The treadmill is a great tool for keeping you on track with your schedule, but it can mess with your rhythmic breathing effort. The digital readouts can begin to dictate your workout, overriding your attention to breathing. I noticed that I would tend to run a bit too fast and work too hard, so I began placing a towel over the digital readout, which then forced me to adjust pace and effort according to how I felt, not according to the numbers on the display. I was back again using rhythmic breathing. Here are a few tips for the treadmill.

- Make sure to follow through on the purpose of your workout.
- Perform a few easy/short runs before you attempt a quality workout.
- Set the incline to 1 percent, which feels more like running outdoors. (Of course, for a hill workout, you will change the inclines according to your workout.)
- Be sure to cool down at the end of your run, and allow the treadmill to come to a complete stop before you step off.

the chapters that follow, approach them as you have your progression to becoming a runner. Keep in mind the most common mistakes that sideline runners—running too fast and/or too far. Do only what feels comfortable for your level of fitness and your lifestyle. If you are eager to move to the next stage of training but don't feel quite ready, repeat your current routine until you feel confident that you are ready to move on. This smart approach to running and training allows you to achieve optimal fitness and performance. It also helps prevent injury and keeps running fun.

Rhythmic Runner:
Leah Zerbe

RUNNER PROFILE: self-proclaimed weekend warrior who enjoys the occasional race
AGE: 30
OCCUPATION: health journalist and farmer

"I don't get side stitches anymore!"

Leah Zerbe could count on getting side stitches almost every time she ran, but she'd run anyway and power on through the pain.

In 2009, Lyme disease sidelined Zerbe from any kind of exercise, but after 2 years of treatment she regained her health and returned to running. "Running is actually part of my treatment," she says. "It helps me keep the Lyme disease under control."

Zerbe had always run on her own, but in spring of 2011 she signed up for Budd Coates's beginning running class. "No one had ever given me any advice about how to breathe during running, and I always used to breathe in through my nose and out through my mouth," she says. In Coates's class, Zerbe learned how to breathe diaphragmatically, how to sync inhalation and exhalation with her footstrikes to optimally manage the impact stress of running, and how to use breathing as a measure of effort.

"I was so out of shape and running was uncomfortable," recalls Zerbe. "The focus on breathing took the focus off of my discomfort. And I don't get side stitches anymore! Honestly, if I hadn't taken Budd's class, I don't know if I'd be running now."

Rhythmic breathing has made running more comfortable in many ways for Zerbe. With a 1-hour commute to the office, fitting in a run is a challenge as Zerbe aims to complete a half-marathon. "I don't train as much as I should," she says, "but I'm still able to do long runs comfortably because of rhythmic breathing. I can use it to stay steady.

"When I'm going up a steep hill with a group of runners, I may not be in front at the bottom, but I'm first or second at the top."

CHAPTER 6

RHYTHMIC BREATHING IN TRAINING

"You play the way you practice."—Glenn "Pop" Warner

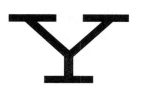ou could head out your front door and run the same route, at the same level of effort, for the same amount of time, day in and day out. If you do so you will become fitter, but eventually your body will adapt to this work. And though you will certainly be able to maintain your fitness, you won't see continued gains. Changing up your runs throughout the week—varying the distance, pace, and terrain—will require that you use your muscles in different ways. This continuously challenges your muscles, improving their performance and ultimately yours as a runner, whether your goal is to run for

personal wellness or to race competitively. Besides, changing it up makes running fun.

Running with Purpose

Jack Daniels, PhD, renowned coach and exercise physiologist, is also famous for remarking, on many occasions, that "every workout should have a purpose." And to achieve that purpose, you need to perform every workout at the appropriate level of effort. Run too hard or too easy and you defeat the purpose. The difficulty comes in monitoring our effort as we run.

Timothy J. Quinn, PhD, associate professor of kinesiology at the University of New Hampshire, and former graduate student Benjamin A. Coons studied exertion during physical activity as it relates to the talk test and other measures of exercise intensity. (See "Measuring Effort in the Lab" on page 73.) Here are their conclusions:

> "One of the most difficult parts of an exercise prescription is the regulation and control of exercise intensity. Pre-established methods of gauging exercise intensity, such as heart rate, [max VO$_2$], and RPE [rate of perceived exertion] are well-established and widely used. However, the intensity prescribed using these methods may be too strenuous for certain populations or may result in an inadequate training stimulus for more conditioned individuals. Identifying a simple method of prescribing exercise intensity to more or less conditioned individuals would be beneficial." (From "The Talk Test and its relationship with the ventilatory and lactate thresholds," *Journal of Sports Sciences*, August 2011)

That simple method of determining the right exercise intensity for each run is rhythmic breathing. Applying it to every run will ensure that you achieve the goal of that run. Following are the different types of workouts you can mix into your training, the purpose of each, and the appropriate rhythmic breathing effort (RBE) for that workout.

The Long Run

The purpose of a long run is to build up your running endurance—to teach your body to maintain effort for a "long" period of time. The length depends on your level of running fitness and your goal, and the distance increases as your training progresses. Long runs train your slow-twitch

Train Like a Kenyan

Prior to the 2012 Olympic Games, *Runner's World* magazine interviewed six former US Olympians about their experience and their training, including Bob Kennedy, a two-time Olympian who in 1996 set the American record for the 5000 meters, a mark that stood until 2009. Here's a piece of what Kennedy shared about running with his Kenyan training partners.

Runner's World: Besides being exposed to faster tempos, what else did you learn from your Kenyan training partners?

Kennedy: One of the biggest things I learned is that sometimes you have to relax. I'll give you an example. Most American athletes run too hard, too often. Recovery days have to be easy. One day in England, I was going out for an easy afternoon 6-mile run with Moses Kiptanui, 3 days before a meet in Stockholm. We jogged the 300 meters to the park and Moses stops and says he's too tired to run and he goes home. I'm wondering if he is okay. Three days later he runs 7:58 for the steeplechase, just missing the world record.

I asked him later about skipping that easy run and he said sometimes his body tells him it's not time to train. Kenyans understand their body better, I think. Whereas a Western athlete, if they are tired, would try to jam their way through it. I learned that from them and was a better athlete as a result.

and intermediate-twitch muscle fibers, making them stronger and better adapted for endurance. (See "The Muscle Mix" on page 76 for a discussion of the three groups of muscle fiber.) Though slow-twitch muscle fibers rule long, slow distance, they will gradually fatigue, and your body will recruit more intermediate-twitch fibers. Running long improves the endurance qualities of those intermediate fibers as well as your body's ability to bring them to the task.

RBE: 51

The effort: Easy throughout the length of the run. You should be able to comfortably hold a conversation through the entire distance and finish feeling tired but not spent. At first, you may need to slow down toward the end of your long run to stay at 51, but as you get fitter, you will be able to maintain the same pace throughout.

Because of the long and easy effort, this run allows you to relax into the rhythm of your running and enjoy that "sweet spot" where you feel like you are indeed running on air and you could run forever.

A word of caution: If your RBE sneaks up to 52 or 53, you will find yourself becoming too fatigued to continue, and you'll need to cut your run short. It will take longer to recover from this run, which will then diminish the quality of subsequent workouts.

The Easy Run

Rest and recovery are your goals for this workout. Any form of exercise, running included, breaks down muscle and bone tissue on a microscopic level, and as your body repairs the damage, it builds stronger, more resilient tissue. You need to give your body time to restore itself. If you run hard every day, your body cannot complete the necessary repairs and you drive damage even further, eventually to the point of injury. By attempting quality runs every day, you actually diminish the quality of your training. You will find it difficult to run the pace or distance you set for yourself, and

Measuring Effort in the Lab

A study conducted at the University of New Hampshire by Timothy J. Quinn, PhD, and Benjamin A. Coons found the talk test to be an effective means of evaluating exercise intensity. The chart below compares data from the study with effort levels from the Rhythmic Breathing Effort Scale. You'll see that the rhythmic breathing efforts align with the talk test as an effective way to monitor exercise intensity as measured by percentage of heart rate and percentage of max VO_2. (For an in-depth explanation of the chart below and the research, see "The Talk Test and its relationship with ventilatory and lactate thresholds," *Journal of Sports Sciences*, August 2011.)

	VARIABLE			
	% MAX VO$_2$	% MAX HR	RATE OF PERCEIVED EXERTION	RHYTHMIC BREATHING EFFORT (RBE)
Ventilatory Threshold	51.2 ± 6.7	77.9 ± 4.8	10.7 ± 1.5	51
Lactate Threshold	65.4 ± 7.1	83.7 ± 5.1	12.5 ± 2.2	52
Last + Talk Test (could talk comfortably)	64.1 ± 4.7	82.4 ± 7.1	11.9 ± 1.8	52
± Talk Test (could not talk comfortably)	70.9 ± 6.5	90.4 ± 5.9	14.8 ± 1.6	53
– Talk Test (could not talk)	78.6 ± 6.9	93.7 ± 4.0	16.3 ± 1.7	31

Notes:

1. Numbers preceded by ± represent significant differences at P50.05.

2. Ventilatory threshold is the point during exercise at which you begin to breathe heavily to rid your body of excess carbon dioxide so that you can take in more oxygen.

3. Lactate threshold is the point at which muscles can no longer metabolize and remove lactic acid produced during exercise.

you'll feel greater fatigue at the end of your workouts and throughout the day. Rest is essential to injury-free running and your best performance in training and racing.

RBE: 0 or 51

The effort: Depending on which running schedule you use (see Chapter 7), the easy run will mean no running at all or a short workout of anywhere from 20 to 40 minutes. The effort for the short runs should be very easy, an RBE of 51. The purpose is to get your blood flowing and muscles moving. You should not feel any fatigue whatsoever during or at the end of your run. For the runner with a minor injury or the runner who is often injured, the easy days are perfect for cross-training to relieve some of the impact stress of running.

The Moderate Run

This run separates the training schedules that you'll find in Chapters 7, 8, and 9 from the conventional hard/easy training method. It acts as a transition from the easy training day to a quality, or hard, day. You spend a bit more time on your feet than you do on an easy run, and you may even include a few strides to open up your stride length and prepare yourself for the next day's quality run.

RBE: 51

The effort: This is an aerobic run at a relaxed effort—a conversational pace. It's the perfect run to take on your local trails. If you want to include some strides, here's how: Warm up with several minutes of running at 51. Pick up your pace to an RBE of 31 for 20 seconds and then drop back down to 51 for 40 seconds. Do 6 to 10 strides, keeping the 20 seconds of speed at an RBE of 31—comfortably fast. The goal of these is to increase the power and length of your stride.

The Hill Run

Running over hilly terrain pushes you into a harder effort without the structure of a measured interval workout. It fits nicely into base training, providing some quality running that helps prepare your body for the harder, faster workouts of race-specific training. If you don't plan to race or race competitively, running hills still offers benefits. It boosts your leg strength and your cardiovascular fitness and brings variety to your running routine. (See Chapter 10 for detailed information on hill training.)

RBE: 51 to 52

The effort: You'll start out on flat terrain, running a relaxed and comfortable 51. As you climb a hill, you'll feel the effort increase to 52, at which point you'll be breathing deeper—you'll still be able to talk but not so easily or comfortably as at an RBE of 51. As you recover coming down a hill, your effort and breathing will relax back to a 51. Try to choose a different course for each of your hill runs, or run the course in the opposite direction to mix things up.

Long Intervals

You can run long intervals on flat or hilly terrain or a combination of both. I have run and coached these workouts on the track, a cinder path, cross-country courses, and rural roads. My current favorite spot is a grass course that I helped develop around a local patch of farmland. It includes a mostly flat loop for 1-kilometer intervals of 3 to 4 minutes in length, another stretch with a nice steady incline of 500 meters to 1 kilometer for long uphill or downhill intervals, and another rolling section for an up-and-down 1-kilometer interval. (In the training schedules I've provided in Chapters 8 and 9, I've identified specific workouts for specific days in the cycle.)

Long intervals develop strength and power. They recruit both your slow-twitch and intermediate-twitch muscle fibers, forcing the slow-twitch fibers to maximum speed of contraction and training the two muscle types to work efficiently together.

The Muscle Mix

Not all muscle is created equal, and the muscle you use to move your body—the skeletal muscle—has three different types of cells, aka muscle fibers. Because those fibers have different specialties, you achieve your best running performance with a mix of workouts designed to train specific groups of muscle fibers to deliver their best. You'll find those workouts in this book. Here's a closer look at the individual groups of muscle fibers and their specialties.

• **Slow-twitch fibers.** No surprise here: This group of muscle cells contracts the slowest of the three. But we love them because they are loaded with mitochondria—organelles where the biochemical processes of respiration and energy production occur—and myoglobin, a protein that stores oxygen. Slow-twitch fibers ensure a steady supply of oxygen and energy, which means they excel in their contribution to aerobic, long-distance running.

• **Fast-twitch fibers.** These contract the fastest and most forcefully of the muscle fiber groups to propel you forward with speed. They have little capacity for carrying oxygen and creating energy, which is of little concern for sprinters who desire maximum speed over races that last seconds.

• **Intermediate-twitch fibers.** This type of muscle falls between slow-twitch and fast-twitch in its capabilities. These fibers carry oxygen and create energy, and they contract faster and more forcefully than slow-twitch fibers but are not as powerful as fast-twitch. They often work in conjunction with slow-twitch fibers during long, slow runs or races and with fast-twitch fibers for faster, shorter distances.

Every skeletal muscle in your body (hamstring, calf, glutes, and so forth) contains all three types of fiber, but the amount of each is determined by your genetics. Top distance runners have a high percentage of slow- and intermediate-twitch fibers, while sprinters' muscles pack lots of fast-twitch. Training won't create more of any of these fiber types, but it can improve their performance and thus yours.

RBE: 31 to 32

The effort: These workouts should feel harder than your easy or moderate runs, similar to the early effort of a 5-K or 10-K race.

The Tempo Run

Similar to long intervals, the tempo run strengthens your slow-twitch and intermediate-twitch muscle fibers but over a longer, sustained effort. It teaches you to maintain a comfortably hard effort for a longer period of time than what you would run for interval training. Perhaps the most beneficial quality of this workout is that it improves your ability to concentrate, stay in the moment, and hold your pace. Occasionally you may substitute a race for this workout.

RBE: 51 and 52

The effort: Think of this workout in thirds: The first third is run at 51, then you up the tempo, running at 52, for the middle third, and finally ease back to 51 for the final third. So, for example, if you were running for 60 minutes, you'd run 20 minutes at 51, 20 minutes at 52, and finish with 20 minutes at 51. The easy thirds recruit your slow-twitch muscle fibers, while the middle third works both your slow-twitch and intermediate-twitch muscle fibers.

Short Intervals

This is the workout that exercises your fast-twitch fibers—the ones with explosive power that give you speed. You have a couple of options: several intervals of 30 to 90 seconds on a flat surface (track, road, grass, or trail) or several 10- to 15-second bursts up a short, steep hill. While the goal is to strengthen your fast-twitch fibers, you will also work intermediate muscle fibers in these workouts and develop greater efficiency in using both types of fiber together.

RBE: 33 or 2:1:1:1

The effort: This workout demands the hardest of your rhythmic breathing efforts. You will run all out on these intervals.

Time Trials

Time trials have been defined a number of different ways by a number of different coaches over the years. With rhythmic breathing training, you use a time trial simply to gauge your improvement. This will be the one training run in which you time your pace over a given distance. Choose a course that you've done several times already in training. Just before you head out, start your watch, but leave it behind. As soon as you return, stop your watch and record your time. Remember, as your fitness improves, your rate of perceived exertion decreases, meaning that as you become fitter, running at 51 will feel more comfortable at a faster pace. So, as your training progresses, your time trials will get faster. Don't forget, however, to take into account the environment—wind, heat, humidity, snow—that you encountered during these time trials because, of course, that affects your effort and pace. Plan these time trials on day 7 or 10 of your workout schedule.

RBE: 51 to 52

The effort: Run at an *honest* 51—an easy, conversation-allowing effort—with the occasional rise in effort to 52 on the inclines.

With these eight types of workouts laid out, the next step is to assign them a place in your training plan. Again, the goals are injury-free running and optimal training for best performance.

Applying RBE to Existing Training Programs

Quite honestly, once you learn rhythmic breathing and can apply the rhythmic breathing efforts (RBEs) to different types of workouts, you can continue training as you always have, use it with programs you've downloaded from Web sites such as Smart Runner or TrainingPeaks, and even apply it to the workouts your coach gives you at practice. The way you apply rhythmic breathing will be the same regardless of the training method. Following are a couple of weeks from Arthur Lydiard's program for marathoners. The first is a typical week during the base training stage. I've included the appropriate rhythmic breathing effort for each workout.

A Warmup for Asthma Sufferers

It's tough to "run on air" when you aren't getting enough. But growing research shows that by strengthening your respiratory muscles (see Chapter 14), using patterned breathing, and performing a proper warmup, an athlete can reduce asthmatic symptoms.

Historically, swimmers experience fewer symptoms of asthma than land athletes do, which may be due to the rhythmic breathing and increased breathing resistance that swimming demands.

If you suffer from asthma, in addition to rhythmic breathing and inspiratory muscle training (IMT), try this simple warmup, which gradually increases the physical stress of running on your pulmonary system:

5-10 minutes @ 51 RBE
10 seconds @ 52 RBE
50 seconds @ 51 RBE
10 seconds @ 52 RBE
50 seconds @ 51 RBE
20 seconds @ 52 RBE
40 seconds @ 51 RBE
20 seconds @ 52 RBE
40 seconds @ 51 RBE
30 seconds @ 52 RBE
1 minute @ 51 RBE
1 minute @ 52 RBE
1 minute @ 51 RBE
2 minutes @ 52 RBE
1 minute @ 51 RBE
3 minutes @ 52 RBE
1 minute @ 51 RBE

DAY	WORKOUT	RBE
Monday	Long aerobic running, 1 hour	51–52
Tuesday	Long aerobic running, 1½ hours	51–52
Wednesday	Easy fartlek* running, 1 hour, on hills	52–31
Thursday	Repeat Tuesday's session	51–52
Friday	Jogging, 1 hour	51
Saturday	Repeat Tuesday's session	51–52

*Fartlek, also called speed play, is when, after a 10-minute warmup at an easy pace, you run unmeasured distances at a variety of paces, mixing easy, moderate, and hard efforts.

Fast-forward to a week halfway through Lydiard's marathon training program (about 8 weeks prior to the marathon):

DAY	WORKOUT	RBE
Monday	1-hour run	51–52
	with 10 to 12 100-meter sprints	31–32
Tuesday	Long aerobic running, 1½ hours	51–52
Wednesday	Time trials, 5-K	32
Thursday	Repeat Tuesday's session	51–52
Friday	Easy fartlek running, ½ hour	51–31
Saturday	Time trials, 25-K	52–31

You can do the same with any training program. Simply use the workout descriptions and rhythmic breathing efforts described at the beginning of this chapter and assign the appropriate RBE to each day's run. Eventually, knowing what RBE is required becomes automatic. Consider the following possible scenarios you might experience in coach-directed workouts.

Scenario 1. Coach says: "Great race yesterday. Let's go easy today."

You think: I need to keep my effort at 51, and if my teammates start to pull away, I'll just let them go.

Scenario 2. Coach says: "Run your warmup down to the trails; do a 3-mile run at tempo and cool down on the way back."

You think: Keep it at 51 to the trails, ease into 52-31, head home at 51.

Scenario 3. Coach says: "We're going to pick it up today. Warm up for 3 miles and meet me at the track for eight 400s with 200-meter recoveries; then you'll do a 3-mile cooldown."

You think: Run 3 miles at 51; the 400s should be at 32 or 33; ease back to 51 on the recoveries; and then it's 51 for the cooldown.

In my own experience, the rhythmic breathing method of training has not only helped me to run mostly injury-free, it has made running so much simpler and has allowed me to fulfill the purpose of my workouts. On an easy run, I can feel when I'm not at an RBE of 51 and I can immediately adjust my effort. If I need to do a long time trial, I know I need to pick up the pace to a level that puts me in the 52-31 breathing effort.

Rhythmic Runner:
Jamie Hibell

RUNNER PROFILE: competitive athlete in high school, college, and postcollege with PRs of 14:47 for 5-K, 1:06:09 for the half, and 2:22:09 for the marathon

AGE: 40

OCCUPATION: high school mathematics teacher; head indoor track/assistant outdoor track coach, Easton Area High School; assistant women's cross-country coach, DeSales University, Center Valley, Pennsylvania

> "I concentrate on my breathing and everything pops back to where it's supposed to be."

Jamie Hibell, the top American finisher at the 2000 Boston Marathon, and Budd Coates had trained together for years.

"Budd had mentioned the benefit of rhythmic breathing for injury prevention," recalls Hibell. "But back then [the late '90s] he was still researching how to incorporate breathing in training." In 2011, Hibell got the whole program.

"I adapted to it pretty easily," he says. "On a run, I can tune in to my breathing effort and know immediately where I'm at. When I'm doing a hard workout, if I find that I'm struggling, I concentrate on my breathing and everything pops back to where it's supposed to be. Everything—my rhythm's back, my running feels smoother and more controlled, my form cleans up."

Hibell teaches rhythmic breathing to the high school runners he coaches, and they have also enjoyed the benefits of focusing on their breathing. (See Tyler Caul's story on page 117.) As for Hibell himself, family, work, and coaching ("I spend more time coaching than I do running") have been somewhat of a hindrance to his competitive career. But at 40, he hungers to compete as a masters runner. And it's a good bet he'll make his mark.

CHAPTER 7

THE 14–DAY TRAINING PLAN

"Great things are not done by impulse, but by a series of small things brought together."

—Vincent Van Gogh

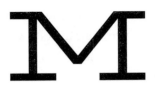ost of the running programs you will find in print or online today follow a 7-day weekly cycle of workouts, which fits very nicely into a 5-day workweek followed by a 2-day weekend but is not ideal for optimal training. A 7-day cycle makes it very hard—if not impossible—to put together a mix of the required components of a successful training program.

Many successful coaches and elite athletes instead use a 9-day cycle made popular by Joe Vigil (who coached Olympian Pat Porter for years). Others follow cycles up to 21 days in length. What's common to these longer cycles is a microcycle of 3 days, which allows you to run a quality workout followed by an easy/recovery day and then a day of moderate running.

The hard-day/easy-day training philosophy, which flourished in the '80s and beyond, had a significant drawback—delayed-onset muscle soreness (DOMS). Research shows that after a bout of hard physical exertion, such as a quality workout or race, muscle soreness peaks 48 hours later. So it is wise to schedule 2 easier days between hard runs. (Although you could sneak in a second quality workout the very next day before DOMS sets in. This was an approach that Arthur Lydiard used with the athletes he coached, and it has been found to be physiologically sound by exercise scientist and running coach Jack Daniels, PhD.)

Because I've always worked full-time during my running career, the 9-day training cycle didn't fit into my workweek, and 21 days was simply too long for me, so I developed a 14-day training cycle. This allowed me four 3-day microcycles, a short turnover day during which I would run some short, fast repeats, and a day off. In addition, I could alter this cycle slightly to include back-to-back days of quality training. Here's the foundation of the 14-day cycle:

The specific run you do each day will depend on a variety of factors: your experience as a runner, your level of fitness, how much mileage you are running, and how much time you have to dedicate. For someone who runs 25 miles a week, an easy day may mean zero mileage. The runner who covers 80 miles in a week may run 4 to 6 miles on an easy day. With that in mind, I have taken the 14-day training cycle and developed four schedules for base training: A, B, C, and D.

I also chose to define runs by time rather than mileage, and there are several reasons for this. First, your body understands effort and distance as it relates to time. It doesn't know miles. The rhythmic breathing method of training is an effort-based system that guides you through both a quality and quantity of effort that will keep you injury-free and help you reach

Basic 14-Day Training Cycle

DAY	WORKOUT
1	Long
2	Easy
3	Moderate
4	Long Intervals
5	Easy
6	Moderate
7	Tempo/Rolling Hills
8	Easy
9	Moderate
10	Long Intervals
11	Easy
12	Moderate
13	Short Speed
14	Zero

your best running performance. To stay on track with this kind of training, it helps to put mileage and pace per mile out of one's mind. Certainly, you will want to do time trials to gauge where your pace is relative to an upcoming race, and you will use races to gauge your fitness and speed for your target goal. But putting forth the appropriate amount and level of effort every day is the most efficient and effective means of fulfilling the purpose of every run and improving your strength and speed.

Running by time and effort means that you will always do the workout you are meant to do on a given day. Consider how the environment affects your running. Let's say you are scheduled to run an easy 30 minutes on a hot and humid day. You head out the door and, with a focus on your breathing, you adjust your pace so that you are running at a rhythmic breathing effort of 51; you maintain that effort, and in 30 minutes you've completed your workout. Now, instead let's say you are scheduled to run an easy 4 miles, which you can usually complete in about 30 minutes. But it's hot and humid. So you either run a comfortable effort and complete your run in more than 30 minutes or you decide you must finish the workout in your usual 30 minutes and run at a harder effort than you should for your easy day. Not only has running by miles cost you more physical effort, it has bruised your psyche by making you aware that you simply couldn't complete those miles at the same effort/pace as you are accustomed to.

Environmental conditions aside, as you get fitter over time, running becomes easier and your pace will naturally increase at a given effort. So that same easy 30-minute run that used to cover 4 miles now covers *more* than 4 miles. But that extra distance doesn't mean you are overextending yourself. It is appropriate, because you are now a stronger runner.

Perhaps the real beauty of defining workouts by time versus miles lies in its simplicity. You know how much *time* you have and you can fit running into the rhythm of your life. You can do these workouts anywhere, anytime. You can step outside and run out for the first 20 minutes of a 40-minute run, then turn around and head home. No need for measured miles or kilometers—there's just you and time and breath.

Four Levels of Training

Following are four schedules for base training—the foundation for all of your running. I assigned workouts to days of the week simply to give you a feel for how this might look on your calendar. Day 1 is the long run in the cycle, so schedule that on the day of the week that you feel will consistently allow you the time to run the distance. For someone who works full-time Monday through Friday, Saturday or Sunday would probably be best. It is essential that you do these workouts in the order listed, but whether day 1 falls on Sunday or Wednesday depends on what works best for your lifestyle. Base training builds your running fitness and prepares you for race-specific training, if that's your goal. Do these runs at a rhythmic breathing effort of 51-52. When you move up to race-specific training, you will be treated to a full menu of intervals, tempo runs, and short speed workouts.

Environmental Impact

Our performance in any physical activity is affected by environmental conditions. As runners, we are never more aware of this than when we line up for a race on a day that is extremely hot and humid. But cold, wind, rain, and terrain all have an impact as well. Sometimes the environment affects the availability of oxygen (high altitude). Other times, environmental conditions (heat and humidity) demand more work from your body, which impacts the distribution of oxygen.

During ideal running weather—cool with low humidity—your body directs bloodflow to your working muscles and away from muscles that are not involved in running. In addition, bloodflow to your digestive system and skin tissue is restricted. Now let's look at what happens when it is hot and humid: Your body needs to prevent overheating by increasing perspiration; therefore, blood is redistributed from your working muscles to your skin. Less oxygen is available to your running muscles, so you either need to breathe more deeply or faster to maintain a particular pace—or you need to slow down.

Rather than concern yourself with pace, with rhythmic breathing you commit yourself to effort. If you are meant to run at an RBE of 51, then that is the effort you put forth whether it is cool and dry or hot and humid. Your pace will follow—faster in cool weather and slower in the heat—but *the effort will feel the same*. When the weather is on the extreme side, and you still intend to attempt your workout, plan on running one RBE lower than what's on your schedule. Or consider taking your workout to the treadmill. (See page 65 for tips on treadmill running.) And remember, there is no shame in canceling a run when environmental conditions place too high a physical demand and a treadmill workout is not an option.

The weather isn't the only factor that influences your running. Lack of sleep, stress, and an oncoming illness can all affect your physical performance. By focusing on rhythmic breathing, you can adjust your running effort to what you are capable of on any given day. And think about what that effort may mean. When your usual pace at 51 feels like a 52 or 53, you need to examine what's going on in your life that is dragging down your physical performance.

SCHEDULE A:
14-Day Training Cycle

DAY	WEEKDAY	RUN (TOTAL MINUTES)
1	Sunday	45–60
2	Monday	0
3	Tuesday	15–20
4	Wednesday	25–30
5	Thursday	0
6	Friday	15–20
7	Saturday	25–30
8	Sunday	0
9	Monday	15–20
10	Tuesday	25–30
11	Wednesday	0
12	Thursday	15–20
13	Friday	15–20
14	Saturday	0

SCHEDULE **B:**
14-Day Training Cycle

DAY	WEEKDAY	RUN (TOTAL MINUTES)
1	Sunday	60–90
2	Monday	0–20
3	Tuesday	30–40
4	Wednesday	40–50
5	Thursday	0–20
6	Friday	30–40
7	Saturday	40–60
8	Sunday	0–20
9	Monday	30–40
10	Tuesday	40–60
11	Wednesday	0–20
12	Thursday	30–40
13	Friday	30–40
14	Saturday	0

SCHEDULE C:
14-Day Training Cycle

DAY	WEEKDAY	RUN (TOTAL MINUTES)
1	Sunday	1½–2 hrs
2	Monday	30–40
3	Tuesday	40–60
4	Wednesday	60–70
5	Thursday	0–30
6	Friday	40–60
7	Saturday	60–70
8	Sunday	0–30
9	Monday	40–60
10	Tuesday	60–70
11	Wednesday	0–30
12	Thursday	40–60
13	Friday	50–60
14	Saturday	0

SCHEDULE **D**:
14-Day Training Cycle

DAY	WEEKDAY	RUN (TOTAL MINUTES)
1	Sunday	2–2½ hours
2	Monday	30–40
3	Tuesday	60–80
4	Wednesday	80–90
5	Thursday	30–40
6	Friday	60–80
7	Saturday	80–90
8	Sunday	0–30
9	Monday	60–80
10	Tuesday	80–90
11	Wednesday	30
12	Thursday	50–60
13	Friday	50–60
14	Saturday	0

Your Best Schedule

Which of the cycles should you choose? If you have completed the beginning running program in Chapter 5, start with Schedule A. Otherwise, think back over your training for the past 2 weeks and add up how much time you've been running; select the schedule that best matches it, keeping in mind that it's always best to err on the conservative side. So if the amount you've been running falls between two levels, choose the easier one.

Complete a schedule at least twice before progressing to the next one. When you feel certain that you can handle more (you should be completing the upper end in the range of recommended workout times for most, if not all, of your runs) and that you have the time and desire to increase the quantity and quality of your running, by all means take on the next challenge. It would serve you best, however, to repeat the same cycle for 1 to 2 months before moving up. That may sound like a long time, but the strength you will gain from adapting to the work will push you to a completely new level of fitness and position you well for the next training challenge. If life causes you to miss a day or two or even three

Racing from Your Base

Though you may not be doing intervals or tempo runs during base training, that doesn't mean you shouldn't run a race—although I'd recommend you not jump into a marathon. Choose anything from 5-K to 10-K. A week before the race, follow the 7-day taper that corresponds to your training schedule (see Chapter 8). And here's a race-day tip: By dividing the race into three stages of effort, you will avoid going out too fast and you'll finish strong.

STAGE	RBE	5-K	10-K
1	52	0-1 mile	0-2 miles
2	52-31	1-2 miles	2-4 miles
3	31-32	2-3.1 miles	4-6.2 miles

of running, simply continue on with whatever you have planned. Don't try to make up the lost workouts. If, however, you miss more than 3 days in a row, or if a couple periods of missed runs occur, repeat the 14-day cycle you are currently running.

Again, the cycles presented here represent base training. They become the foundation of the race-specific training schedules you'll find in the next couple of chapters. But if you want to inject a touch of speedwork into this base training, you can add strides to your runs on days 1, 4, 7, and 10. You'll do these in the middle of your workout after you've warmed up with several minutes at an RBE of 51. Pick up your pace to an RBE of 31 for 20 seconds and then drop back to 51 for 40 seconds; repeat for a total of 6 to 10 strides. Make sure the 20 seconds of speed doesn't sneak up to an effort of 32 or 33. Remember, 31 is the easiest of your speed gears. It should feel comfortably hard. My rule for controlling the pace is that as soon as I feel fast and frisky, I back off. The goal of these is to increase the power and length of your stride, and adding this element to your workouts builds a strong bridge from base training to race training.

Rhythmic Runner:
Kari Dougan

RUNNER PROFILE: a once-competitive runner, who now runs for fitness

AGE: 53

OCCUPATION: fitness instructor and personal trainer

> "The first half-marathon I ran after using rhythmic breathing in training was the most comfortable in my life. And I ran it 30 seconds per mile faster than my previous half!"

Kari Dougan admits that she didn't pay any attention to her breath until she was out of it. "I ran with a lot of serious runners and no one ever talked about breathing," she says. Then she spoke with Budd Coates about a nagging injury in her left hip and about how she could get faster. Coates explained his rhythmic breathing method. And Dougan listened.

"I had trouble finishing speed-work. Rhythmic breathing helped me control my pace so I could do more," she says. And it smoothed out her long runs, too. "I could go 15 miles using rhythmic breathing and not feel winded or fatigued

at the end." The training benefit paid off at the races.

"The first half-marathon I ran after using rhythmic breathing in training was the most comfortable in my life," she says. "And I ran it 30 seconds per mile faster than my previous half!"

And that injury in her left hip? Gone.

With results like these, Dougan eagerly passes on her knowledge of rhythmic breathing to running partners and to the individuals she's trained to run. "They enjoy running more because they are more comfortable doing it," she says. "Now they won't run any other way." And neither will Kari Dougan.

CHAPTER 8

THE 5-K TO THE 10-K

"Success is simple. Do what's right, the right way, at the right time."—Arnold Glasow

T he 5-K—3.1 miles—welcomes everyone. A new runner can participate in a 5-K after completing my beginning running program, with no race-specific training required. The allure for the experienced runner is short speed. The 5-K is the sprint of the distance races. But this race distance is relatively young. Years ago, the 10-K (6.2 miles) was the only option for a runner's first competition—a formidable challenge for anyone new to running. Sometime in the late '80s, 5-Ks began to pop up everywhere, and by the mid-'90s they had started to outnumber 10-Ks. And with good reason, since the longer race places greater demands on both runners and race directors. But as with most trends, what goes out eventually comes back in, and the 10-K is enjoying a resurgence both out of nostalgia for the forgotten distance and, more practically, because it offers a good stepping-stone to longer races.

Because the 5-K and 10-K are short distances, the focus of training skews toward short, fast workouts to develop speed and away from longer, slower running for endurance. Don't get me wrong—endurance is essential to racing the 5-K and 10-K. In fact, it is precisely the balance of speed and endurance that makes these races so challenging.

The only differences between 5-K and 10-K training are the length of the long run and the tempo runs. When you are preparing for a 10-K, run the high end of the distance range given for each workout. For the 5-K, any distance in the range works in your training.

The schedules that follow build from the identically labeled base training schedules in Chapter 7, so if you've been following base Schedule A, you'll move to training Schedule A to prepare for your race. The difference in these schedules is that quality workouts—long intervals, short intervals, and tempo runs—have been added to the race training cycles. It's best to spend as many weeks as possible running your base miles before embarking on race-specific training. When you get hungry to compete, target a race that gives you 13 weeks of preparation—12 for training and 1 week to taper before race day.

Each schedule that follows consists of six cycles (remember, each cycle covers 14 days). And they become more challenging in distance, time, and quality as you move up from A to B to C to D. If your goal is to improve your race performance to your fullest potential, you will want to progress in this order through base training and then race-specific training. Let's say you've raced off training Schedule A. Next, move up your base training to Schedule B and follow with the level B race-specific cycles.

Perhaps, however, the demands of your life don't allow you the extra time required of Schedule B. In that case, try to move up in quality—run the B workouts given for days 1, 4, 7, 10, and 13 first in base training and then in race-specific training. While working full-time during my competitive days, I used a similar strategy.

Keep in mind that the core goal of this book is to teach you to run from within, to develop the mind-body connection that allows you to manage your ability and physiology optimally for your best performance. That same principle applies to the broader design of your life. You have only so much physical and mental energy to give. You need to think about what is the right amount of energy to give to running and racing—the right place for it in your life? Rhythmic running also aims to fit running into the rhythm of your whole life.

Now choose your plan and let's get started.

SCHEDULE **A**: 5–K TO 10–K
Cycles 1 and 2 (weeks 1 through 4)

DAY	WEEKDAY	WORKOUT	RUN (DISTANCE @ RBE)	
1	Sunday	long run	45–60 min @ 51	
2	Monday	easy	0	
3	Tuesday	moderate	15–20 min @ 51	
4	Wednesday	long intervals	10 min @ 51	
			2 min @ 31 2 min @ 51	run 3 times
			5–10 min @ 51	
5	Thursday	easy	0	
6	Friday	moderate	15–20 min @ 51	
7	Saturday	tempo	10 min @ 51 10 min @ 52 10 min @ 51	
8	Sunday	easy	0	
9	Monday	moderate	15–20 min @ 51	
10	Tuesday	long intervals	10 min @ 51 3 min @ 31 3 min @ 51 3 min @ 31 10 min @ 51	
11	Wednesday	easy	0	
12	Thursday	moderate	15–20 min @ 51	
13	Friday	short intervals	5 min @ 51	
			1 min @ 32 1 min @ 51	run 5 times
			5 min @ 51	
14	Saturday	zero	0	

SCHEDULE **A**: 5-K TO 10-K
Cycles 3 and 4 (weeks 5 through 8)

DAY	WEEKDAY	WORKOUT	RUN (DISTANCE @ RBE)	
1	Sunday	long run	60–70 min @ 51	
2	Monday	easy	0	
3	Tuesday	moderate	15–20 min @ 51	
4	Wednesday	long intervals	10 min @ 51	
			2 min @ 31 2 min @ 51	run 3 times
			5–10 min @ 51	
5	Thursday	easy	0	
6	Friday	moderate	15–20 min @ 51	
7	Saturday	tempo	10 min @ 51 10 min @ 52-31 10 min @ 51	
8	Sunday	easy	0	
9	Monday	moderate	15–20 min @ 51	
10	Tuesday	long intervals	10 min @ 51 3 min @ 32 3 min @ 51 3 min @ 32 10 min @ 51	
11	Wednesday	easy	0	
12	Thursday	moderate	15–20 min @ 51	
13	Friday	short intervals	5 min @ 51	
			30 sec @ 32 1 min @ 51	run 5 to 7 times
			5 min @ 51	
14	Saturday	zero	0	

SCHEDULE **A**: 5–K TO 10–K
Cycles 5 and 6 (weeks 9 through 12)

DAY	WEEKDAY	WORKOUT	RUN (DISTANCE @ RBE)	
1	Sunday	long run	60–80 min @ 51	
2	Monday	easy	0	
3	Tuesday	moderate	15–20 min @ 51	
4	Wednesday	long intervals	10 min @ 51 1 min @ 32 1 min @ 51 2 min @ 32 2 min @ 51 3 min @ 31 5–10 min @ 51	
5	Thursday	easy	0	
6	Friday	moderate	15–20 min @ 51	
7	Saturday	tempo	10 min @ 51 5 min @ 31 1 min @ 51 4 min @ 31 10 min @ 51	
8	Sunday	easy	0	
9	Monday	moderate	15–20 min @ 51	
10	Tuesday	long intervals	10 min @ 51 3 min @ 32 2 min @ 51 3 min @ 32 10 min @ 51	
11	Wednesday	easy	0	
12	Thursday	moderate	15–20 min @ 51	
13	Friday	short intervals	5 min @ 51	
			30 sec @ 33 1 min @ 51 1 min @ 33 1 min @ 51	run 2 or 3 times
			5 min @ 51	
14	Saturday	zero	0	

SCHEDULE **A**: 5-K TO 10-K
Taper and Recovery
(days leading up to and following the race)

DAY	WEEKDAY	RUN (DISTANCE @ RBE)	
1	Sunday	25–30 min @ 51	
2	Monday	0	
3	Tuesday	15–20 min @ 51	
4	Wednesday	5 min @ 51	
		1 min @ 31 1 min @ 51	run 2 or 3 times
		5 min @ 51	
5	Thursday	0	
6	Friday	0–10 min @ 51	
7	Saturday	10–15 min @ 51	
8	Sunday	5 min @ 51 **RACE** 5 min @ 51 or walk	
9	Monday	0	
10	Tuesday	0	
11	Wednesday	15–20 min @ 51	
12	Thursday	0	
13	Friday	5 min @ 51	
		30 sec @ 52 1 min @ 51	repeat 2 or 3 times
		5 min @ 51	
14	Saturday	0	

SCHEDULE **B**: 5-K TO 10-K
Cycles 1 and 2 (weeks 1 through 4)

DAY	WEEKDAY	WORKOUT	RUN (DISTANCE @ RBE)	
1	Sunday	long run	60–90 min @ 51	
2	Monday	easy	0–20 min @ 51	
3	Tuesday	moderate	30–40 min @ 51	
4	Wednesday	long intervals	10–15 min @ 51	
			3 min @ 31 3 min @ 51	run 4 to 8 times
			10–15 min @ 51	
5	Thursday	easy	0–20 min @ 51	
6	Friday	moderate	30–40 min @ 51	
7	Saturday	tempo	10–15 min @ 51 10 min @ 52 3 min @ 51 10 min @ 52	
			3 min @ 51 10 min @ 52	optional
			10 min @ 51	
8	Sunday	easy	0–20 min @ 51	
9	Monday	moderate	30–40 min @ 51	
10	Tuesday	long intervals	10–15 min @ 51 2 min @ 31 2 min @ 51 3 min @ 31 3 min @ 51 4 min @ 31 10–15 min @ 51	
11	Wednesday	easy	0–20 min @ 51	
12	Thursday	moderate	30–40 min @ 51	
13	Friday	short intervals	10 min @ 51	
			1 min @ 32 1 min @ 51	run 5 to 10 times
			10 min @ 51	
14	Saturday	zero	0	

SCHEDULE **B**: 5–K TO 10–K
Cycle 3 (weeks 5 and 6)

DAY	WEEKDAY	WORKOUT	RUN (DISTANCE @ RBE)	
1	Sunday	long run	60–90 min @ 51	
2	Monday	easy	0–20 min @ 51	
3	Tuesday	moderate	30–40 min @ 51	
4	Wednesday	long intervals	10–15 min @ 51	
			4 min @ 31 4 min @ 51	run 3 to 5 times
			10–15 min @ 51	
5	Thursday	easy	0–20 min @ 51	
6	Friday	moderate	30–40 min @ 51	
7	Saturday	tempo	10–15 min @ 51 15 min @ 52 5 min @ 51 15 min @ 52 10–15 min @ 51	
8	Sunday	easy	0–20 min @ 51	
9	Monday	moderate	30–40 min @ 51	
10	Tuesday	long intervals	10–15 min @ 51 2 min @ 31 2 min @ 51 3 min @ 31 3 min @ 51 4 min @ 31 10–15 min @ 51	
11	Wednesday	easy	0–20 min @ 51	
12	Thursday	moderate	30–40 min @ 51	
13	Friday	short intervals	10 min @ 51	
			30 sec @ 32 1 min @ 51	run 7 to 12 times
			10 min @ 51	
14	Saturday	zero	0	

SCHEDULE **B**: 5-K TO 10-K
Cycle 4 (weeks 7 and 8)

DAY	WEEKDAY	WORKOUT	RUN (DISTANCE @ RBE)		
1	Sunday	long run	60–90 min @ 51		
2	Monday	easy	0–20 min @ 51		
3	Tuesday	moderate	30–40 min @ 51		
4	Wednesday	long intervals	10–15 min @ 51		
			5 min @ 31 4 min @ 51	run 2 or 3 times	
			10–15 min @ 51		
5	Thursday	easy	0–20 min @ 51		
6	Friday	moderate	30–40 min @ 51		
7	Saturday	tempo	10–15 min @ 51 20 min @ 52 5 min @ 51 10 min @ 52 10–15 min @ 51		
8	Sunday	easy	0–20 min @ 51		
9	Monday	moderate	30–40 min @ 51		
10	Tuesday	long intervals	10–15 min @ 51 4 min @ 31 3 min @ 51 3 min @ 31 2 min @ 51 2 min @ 32 1 min @ 51 1 min @ 32 10–15 min @ 51		
11	Wednesday	easy	0–20 min @ 51		
12	Thursday	moderate	30–40 min @ 51		
13	Friday	short intervals	10 min @ 51		
			1 min @ 32 1 min @ 51	run 7 to 12 times	
			10 min @ 51		
14	Saturday	zero	0		

SCHEDULE **B**: 5-K TO 10-K
Cycles 5 and 6 (weeks 9 through 12)

DAY	WEEKDAY	WORKOUT	RUN (DISTANCE @ RBE)		
1	Sunday	long run	60–90 min @ 51		
2	Monday	easy	0–20 min @ 51		
3	Tuesday	moderate	30–40 min @ 51		
4	Wednesday	long intervals	10–15 min @ 51		
			6 min @ 31 3 min @ 51	run 3 or 4 times	
			10–15 min @ 51		
5	Thursday	easy	0–20 min @ 51		
6	Friday	moderate	30–40 min @ 51		
7	Saturday	tempo	10–15 min @ 51 25–30 min @ 52 10–15 min @ 51		
8	Sunday	easy	0–20 min @ 51		
9	Monday	moderate	30–40 min @ 51		
10	Tuesday	long intervals	10–15 min @ 51 4 min @ 31 3 min @ 51 3 min @ 31 2 min @ 51 2 min @ 31 10–15 min @ 51		
11	Wednesday	easy	0–20 min @ 51		
12	Thursday	moderate	30–40 min @ 51		
13	Friday	short intervals	10 min @ 51		
			1 min @ 32 1 min @ 51	run twice	complete entire cycle twice
			30 sec @ 32 1 min @ 51	run twice	
			10 min @ 51		
14	Saturday	zero	0		

SCHEDULE **B**: 5–K TO 10–K
Taper and Recovery
(days leading up to and following the race)

DAY	WEEKDAY	RUN (DISTANCE @ RBE)	
1	Sunday	40–50 min @ 51	
2	Monday	0	
3	Tuesday	20–30 @ 51	
4	Wednesday	10 min @ 51	
		1 min @ 31 1 min @ 51 1½ min @ 31 1½ min @ 51	run 2 or 3 times
		10 min @ 51	
5	Thursday	0–15 min @ 51	
6	Friday	0	
7	Saturday	15–20 min @ 51	
8	Sunday	10–15 min @ 51 **RACE** 10–15 min @ 51	
9	Monday	0–20 min @ 51	
10	Tuesday	20–30 min @ 51	
11	Wednesday	0–20 min @ 51	
12	Thursday	30–40 min @ 51	
13	Friday	10 min @ 51	
		30 sec @ 31 30 sec @ 51	run 10 to 15 times
		10 min @ 51	
14	Saturday	0	

SCHEDULE **C**: 5–K TO 10–K
Cycles 1 and 2 (weeks 1 through 4)

DAY	WEEKDAY	WORKOUT	RUN (DISTANCE @ RBE)	
1	Sunday	long	1½–2 hrs @ 51	
2	Monday	easy	30–40 min @ 51	
3	Tuesday	moderate	40–60 min @ 51	
4	Wednesday	long intervals	15–20 min @ 51	
			6 min @ 31 4 min @ 51	run 3 to 6 times
			15–20 min @ 51	
5	Thursday	easy	0–30 min @ 51	
6	Friday	moderate	40–60 min @ 51	
7	Saturday	long intervals	15–20 min @ 51 10 min @ 52 2 min @ 51 8 min @ 52 2 min @ 51 6 min @ 52 15–20 min @ 51	
8	Sunday	easy	0–30 min @ 51	
9	Monday	moderate	40–60 min @ 51	
10	Tuesday	long intervals	15–20 min @ 51	
			4 min @ 31 3 min @ 51	run 3 to 8 times
			15–20 min @ 51	
11	Wednesday	easy	0–30 min @ 51	
12	Thursday	moderate	40–60 min @ 51	
13	Friday	short intervals	10 min @ 51	
			1 min @ 32 1 min @ 51	run 10 to 15 times
			10 min @ 51	
14	Saturday	zero	0	

SCHEDULE C: 5–K TO 10–K
Cycles 3 and 4 (weeks 5 through 8)

DAY	WEEKDAY	WORKOUT	RUN (DISTANCE @ RBE)	
1	Sunday	long	1½–2 hrs @ 51	
2	Monday	easy	30–40 min @ 51	
3	Tuesday	moderate	40–60 min @ 51	
4	Wednesday	long intervals	15–20 min @ 51	
			7 min @ 31 3 min @ 51	run 3 to 6 times
			15–20 min @ 51	
5	Thursday	easy	0–30 min @ 51	
6	Friday	moderate	40–60 min @ 51	
7	Saturday	long intervals	15–20 min @ 51 10 min @ 52 2 min @ 51 10 min @ 52 2 min @ 51 10 min @ 52 15–20 min @ 51	
8	Sunday	easy	0–30 min @ 51	
9	Monday	moderate	40–60 min @ 51	
10	Tuesday	long intervals	15–20 min @ 51	
			3 min @ 31 2 min @ 51 4 min @ 31 2 min @ 51	run 2 to 6 times
			15–20 min @ 51	
11	Wednesday	easy	0–30 min @ 51	
12	Thursday	moderate	40–60 min @ 51	
13	Friday	short intervals	10 min @ 51	
			1 min @ 32 1 min @ 51 30 sec @ 32 1 min @ 51	run 7 to 10 times
			10 min @ 51	
14	Saturday	zero	0	

SCHEDULE **C**: 5-K TO 10-K
Cycle 5 (weeks 9 and 10)

DAY	WEEKDAY	WORKOUT	RUN (DISTANCE @ RBE)		
1	Sunday	long	1½–2 hrs @ 51		
2	Monday	easy	30–40 min @ 51		
3	Tuesday	moderate	40–60 min @ 51		
4	Wednesday	long intervals	15–20 min @ 51		
			6 min @ 31 2 min @ 51	run 3 to 6 times	
			15–20 min @ 51		
5	Thursday	easy	0–30 min @ 51		
6	Friday	moderate	40–60 min @ 51		
7	Saturday	long intervals	15–20 min @ 51 15 min @ 52 2 min @ 51 15 min @ 52 15–20 min @ 51		
8	Sunday	easy	0–30 min @ 51		
9	Monday	moderate	40–60 min @ 51		
10	Tuesday	long intervals	15–20 min @ 51		
			4 min @ 31 3 min @ 51 3 min @ 32 2 min @ 51 2 min @ 32 2 min @ 51	run 2 or 3 times	
			15–20 min @ 51		
11	Wednesday	easy	0–30 min @ 51		
12	Thursday	moderate	40–60 min @ 51		
13	Friday	short intervals	10 min @ 51		
			30 sec @ 32 1 min @ 51 1 min @ 32 1 min @ 51 1½ min @ 32 4 min @ 51	run 3 to 5 times	
			10 min @ 51		
14	Saturday	zero	0		

SCHEDULE **C**: 5–K TO 10–K
Cycle 6 (weeks 11 and 12)

DAY	WEEKDAY	WORKOUT	RUN (DISTANCE @ RBE)	
1	Sunday	long	$1^{1}/_{2}$–2 hrs @ 51	
2	Monday	easy	30–40 min @ 51	
3	Tuesday	moderate	40–60 min @ 51	
4	Wednesday	long intervals	15–20 min @ 51	
			4 min @ 31/32 2 min @ 51	run 4 to 8 times
			15–20 min @ 51	
5	Thursday	easy	0–30 min @ 51	
6	Friday	moderate	40–60 min @ 51	
7	Saturday	long intervals	15–20 min @ 51 30 min @ 52 15 min @ 51	
8	Sunday	easy	0–30 min @ 51	
9	Monday	moderate	40–60 min @ 51	
10	Tuesday	long intervals	15–20 min @ 51	
			$1^{1}/_{2}$ min @ 31/32 $1^{1}/_{2}$ min @ 51 3 min @ 31/32 3 min @ 51 $1^{1}/_{2}$ min @ 31/32 2 min @ 51	run 3 to 5 times
			15–20 min @ 51	
11	Wednesday	easy	0–30 min @ 51	
12	Thursday	moderate	40–60 min @ 51	
13	Friday	short intervals	10 min @ 51	
			30 sec @ 32 30 sec @ 51	run 15 to 20 times
			10 min @ 51	
14	Saturday	zero	0	

SCHEDULE **C**: 5-K TO 10-K
Taper and Recovery
(days leading up to and following the race)

DAY	WEEKDAY	RUN (DISTANCE @ RBE)	
1	Sunday	60–80 min @ 51	
2	Monday	0	
3	Tuesday	30–40 min @ 51	
4	Wednesday	15–20 min @ 51	
		$1\frac{1}{2}$ min @ 31 $1\frac{1}{2}$ min @ 51	run 6 to 10 times
		15–20 min @ 51	
5	Thursday	15–20 min @ 51	
6	Friday	0	
7	Saturday	15–20 min @ 51	
8	Sunday	15–20 min @ 51 **RACE** 10–15 min @ 51	
9	Monday	20–30 min @ 51	
10	Tuesday	30–40 min @ 51	
11	Wednesday	20–30 min @ 51	
12	Thursday	30–40 min @ 51	
13	Friday	15–20 min @ 51	
		1 min @ 31 1 min @ 51	run 8 to 12 times
		15–20 min @ 51	
14	Saturday	0	

SCHEDULE **D**: 5–K TO 10–K
Cycles 1 and 2 (weeks 1 through 4)

DAY	WEEKDAY	WORKOUT	RUN (DISTANCE @ RBE)	
1	Sunday	long	$1^1/_2$–2 hrs @ 51	
2	Monday	easy	30–40 min @ 51	
3	Tuesday	moderate	60–80 min @ 51	
4	Wednesday	long intervals	15–20 min @ 51	
			6 min @ 31 4 min @ 51	run 3 to 6 times
			15–20 min @ 51	
5	Thursday	easy	30–40 min @ 51	
6	Friday	moderate	60–80 min @ 51	
7	Saturday	long intervals	15–20 min @ 51 10 min @ 52 2 min @ 51 8 min @ 52 2 min @ 51 6 min @ 52 15–20 min @ 51	
8	Sunday	easy	0–30 min @ 51	
9	Monday	moderate	60–80 min @ 51	
10	Tuesday	long intervals	15–20 min @ 51	
			4 min @ 31 3 min @ 51	run 3 to 8 times
			15–20 min @ 51	
11	Wednesday	easy	30 min @ 51	
12	Thursday	moderate	50–60 min @ 51	
13	Friday	short intervals	10 min @ 51	
			1 min @ 32 1 min @ 51	run 10 to 15 times
			10 min @ 51	
14	Saturday	zero	0	

SCHEDULE **D**: 5-K TO 10-K
Cycles 3 and 4 (weeks 5 through 8)

DAY	WEEKDAY	WORKOUT	RUN (DISTANCE @ RBE)	
1	Sunday	long	1½–2 hrs @ 51	
2	Monday	easy	30–40 min @ 51	
3	Tuesday	moderate	60–80 min @ 51	
4	Wednesday	long intervals	15–20 min @ 51	
			7 min @ 31 3 min @ 51	run 3 to 6 times
			15–20 min @ 51	
5	Thursday	easy	30–40 min @ 51	
6	Friday	moderate	60–80 min @ 51	
7	Saturday	long intervals	15–20 min @ 51 10 min @ 52 2 min @ 51 10 min @ 52 2 min @ 51 10 min @ 52 15–20 min @ 51	
8	Sunday	easy	0–30 min @ 51	
9	Monday	moderate	60–80 min @ 51	
10	Tuesday	long intervals	15–20 min @ 51	
			3 min @ 31 2 min @ 51 4 min @ 31 2 min @ 51	run 2 to 6 times
			15–20 min @ 51	
11	Wednesday	easy	30 min @ 51	
12	Thursday	moderate	50–60 min @ 51	
13	Friday	short intervals	10 min @ 51	
			1 min @ 32 1 min @ 51 30 sec @ 32 1 min @ 51	run 7 to 10 times
			10 min @ 51	
14	Saturday	zero	0	

SCHEDULE **D**: 5-K TO 10-K
Cycle 5 (weeks 9 and 10)

DAY	WEEKDAY	WORKOUT	RUN (DISTANCE @ RBE)	
1	Sunday	long	1½–2 hrs @ 51	
2	Monday	easy	30–40 min @ 51	
3	Tuesday	moderate	60–80 min @ 51	
4	Wednesday	long intervals	15–20 min @ 51	
			6 min @ 31 2 min @ 51	run 3 to 6 times
			15–20 min @ 51	
5	Thursday	easy	30–40 min @ 51	
6	Friday	moderate	60–80 min @ 51	
7	Saturday	long intervals	15–20 min @ 51 15 min @ 52 2 min @ 51 15 min @ 52 15–20 min @ 51	
8	Sunday	easy	0–30 min @ 51	
9	Monday	moderate	60–80 min @ 51	
10	Tuesday	long intervals	15–20 min @ 51	
			4 min @ 31 3 min @ 51 3 min @ 32 2 min @ 51 2 min @ 32 2 min @ 51	run 2 to 3 times
			15–20 min @ 51	
11	Wednesday	easy	30 min @ 51	
12	Thursday	moderate	50–60 min @ 51	
13	Friday	short intervals	10 min @ 51	
			30 sec @ 32 1 min @ 51 1 min @ 32 1 min @ 51 1½ min @ 32 4 min @ 51	run 3 to 5 times
			10 min @ 51	
14	Saturday	zero	0	

SCHEDULE **D**: 5-K TO 10-K
Cycle 6 (weeks 11 and 12)

DAY	WEEKDAY	WORKOUT	RUN (DISTANCE @ RBE)	
1	Sunday	long	1$^{1}/_{2}$–2 hrs @ 51	
2	Monday	easy	30–40 min @ 51	
3	Tuesday	moderate	60–80 min @ 51	
4	Wednesday	long intervals	15–20 min @ 51	
			4 min @ 31/32 2 min @ 51	run 4 to 8 times
			15–20 min @ 51	
5	Thursday	easy	30–40 min @ 51	
6	Friday	moderate	60–80 min @ 51	
7	Saturday	long intervals	15–20 min @ 51 30 min @ 52 15 min @ 51	
8	Sunday	easy	0–30 min @ 51	
9	Monday	moderate	60–80 min @ 51	
10	Tuesday	long intervals	15–20 min @ 51	
			1$^{1}/_{2}$ min @ 31/32 1$^{1}/_{2}$ min @ 51 3 min @ 31/32 3 min @ 51 1$^{1}/_{2}$ min @ 31/32 2 min @ 51	run 3 to 5 times
			15–20 min @ 51	
11	Wednesday	easy	30 min @ 51	
12	Thursday	moderate	50–60 min @ 51	
13	Friday	short intervals	10 min @ 51	
			30 sec @ 32 30 sec @ 51	run 15 to 20 times
			10 min @ 51	
14	Saturday	zero	0	

SCHEDULE **D**: 5-K TO 10-K Taper and Recovery
(days leading up to and following the race)

DAY	WEEKDAY	RUN (DISTANCE @ RBE)	
1	Sunday	60–90 min @ 51	
2	Monday	0–30 min @ 51	
3	Tuesday	40–50 min @ 51	
4	Wednesday	15–20 min @ 51	
		1½ min @ 31 1½ min @ 51	run 6 to 10 times
		15–20 min @ 51	
5	Thursday	20–30 min @ 51	
6	Friday	0	
7	Saturday	20 min @ 51	
8	Sunday	15–20 min @ 51 **RACE** 10–15 min @ 51	
9	Monday	20–40 min @ 51	
10	Tuesday	40–50 min @ 51	
11	Wednesday	20–30 min @ 51	
12	Thursday	30–40 min @ 51	
13	Friday	15–20 min @ 51	
		1 min @ 31 1 min @ 51	run 8 to 12 times
		15–20 min @ 51	
14	Saturday	0	

Rhythmic Runner:
Tyler Caul

RUNNER PROFILE: competitive collegiate runner who specializes in the 800 and 1500 meters

AGE: 19

OCCUPATION: college student

> "With rhythmic breathing, I can keep myself relaxed, and racing is definitely more fun."

In his senior year of high school, Tyler Caul had upped his race pace. But with that new speed came a new pain in his left knee.

Neither doctors nor coaches were able to figure out the cause of the pain, so Caul's high school coach, Jamie Hibell, videotaped Caul running. They discovered that his faster pace had changed his form. He tended to lean back—a sign that his core wasn't strong enough to hold him more upright. He was overstriding, and he was running in a breathing pattern that forced him to always strike the ground with his left foot at the moment when the impact stress of running is greatest. Hibell determined the knee pain was related to a strain in the iliotibial band. He gave Caul some stretches to do and, as a veteran of the rhythmic breathing method (see Hibell's story, page 82), he recommended Caul give it a try, too.

"I couldn't get the breathing patterns down at first," says Caul.

"I was so accustomed *not* to think about breathing as I ran." But he kept working at it, and now rhythmic breathing works for him. The knee pain that plagued him for more than a year is gone, and he's enjoying faster and more comfortable racing.

"Instead of focusing solely on my competitors, I focus on breathing," says Caul. "It keeps me relaxed. Before, as I'd head into the final 200 of an 800-meter race, I would feel like I was hyperventilating. I'd overstride and my upper body would tighten up. It would feel like my shoulders were up to my ears. With rhythmic breathing, I can keep myself relaxed, and racing is definitely more fun."

And more successful, too. While at home and training with Hibell, Caul participated in some USA Track and Field meets and saw improvement in his times for both the 800 and 1500 meters. In the spring of 2013, Caul headed to Shippensburg University.

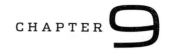

THE 15-K TO THE MARATHON

"We are different, in essence, from other men. If you want to win something, run 100 meters. If you want to experience something, run a marathon." —Emil Zatopek

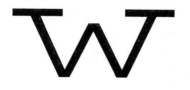hy would anyone want to run, not to mention race, 9, 13, or 26.2 miles? Because the challenge excites us. Sport is about exploiting our physical ability, discovering our physical limits. Every race is a game of speed and endurance, a test to see how long one can sustain a given pace and effort. At the 5-K level, the game tilts toward

how fast you can cover the course. For the 15-K and beyond, the play lies in how long you can maintain your pace. These problems are the same yet not the same.

Longer distances push the boundaries of our endurance. One of my favorites is a 15-K (9.1 miles)—the Berwick Run for the Diamonds. Founded in 1908, it's one of the oldest races in the country and climbs about 500 feet in elevation over the first 4 miles. Though you don't hear much about the 15-K, it's been around for a long time. The half-marathon (13.1 miles), on the other hand, was rare until it became an alternative to the marathon in the late '80s and became a must-run distance before one attempts to complete a full marathon. Interestingly, before the mid-'80s, the first-time marathoner jumped straight from the 10-K to the 26.2-mile marathon distance.

The 15-K and half-marathon and any distance in between have more similarities than differences when it comes to training. The schedules presented later in this chapter will work for all of these distances; I've indicated specific tweaks where appropriate. The key to successful training when moving up is to increase your long run. I also suggest creating a course for your long run that mimics the terrain—hills, loop, out-and-back, road, trail—of your goal race. Teaching your body to adapt to the type of course you'll be running is almost as important as the length of your long run. The more lofty your goals are for your race performance, the more changes you will need to make to the other quality workouts in your schedule to further improve your running fitness.

The Marathon: 26.2 Miles

The marathon will push you to the painful edge of your endurance—yet it seduces. Oh, the glory in conquering this, the most imposing of long-distance races for most of us. To accept the challenge of months of preparation. To overcome the pounding, the persistence, and the pull of those miles to take you down. To venture past the proverbial wall at 20 miles and enter the undiscovered beyond. And finally, to reach across the finish, spent but still whole. It is to become, if just for that moment, just for yourself, a hero.

Many runners approach the marathon as a once-in-a-lifetime goal. The truth is, most of those same runners go on to run a second, a third, maybe a fourth. To quote Frank Shorter: "You need to forget about your last marathon before you start thinking about your next." While I completely agree with Frank, often it's the memory of that last one that inspires you to run another. Perhaps you know you can run it faster next time, or you liked how that rigorous training brought you to a level of incredible fitness. There are perks to the marathon—it is a catalyst to travel, to meet new people, and to expand one's horizons.

The training begins in much the same way as it does for the 15-K or half-marathon, but for the marathon you must increase your long runs. This can be the only change you make to your training, but you must do it. If, based on your past race experiences, you are eyeing a particular marathon time, you'll need to add quality to your training as well, which I've prescribed in the schedules later in this chapter. Keep in mind that come race day, your performance in the marathon, more so than any other race distance, will depend on the weather. If race conditions break unfavorably but you pay close attention to your rhythmic breathing effort and spread that effort out appropriately, you may not run your best race ever but you will run the best race you could on that particular day.

The Training Schedules

As with the 5-K/10-K training programs, you'll find four levels of schedules here: A, B, C, and D, which build from the equivalent base training plans. Each schedule consists of six 14-day cycles for a total of 12 weeks of training to ready you to race anything from the 15-K to the half-marathon.

You will add another three cycles—6 more weeks of training—to get ready for the full marathon.

The path to improvement begins with base training. You must advance in your base training before you move up in race training. So if you've been training and racing at level A, move up to Schedule B in base training for a minimum of 4 weeks, preferably longer, and then you can bump up your race-specific training to Schedule B.

Schedule A: 15-K to Half-Marathon

As with all of the training schedules in this book, day 1 is your long run or endurance workout, and you must run it at a rhythmic breathing effort of 51 for the duration. Over the 12 weeks of training, the length of this run will increase to 2 hours. At that point you should be able to cover 8 miles if you are training for a 15-K and 12 miles if you are training for a half-marathon. If you don't think you will be able to run that far in 2 hours, estimate how much time you think it will take and adjust all of your runs upward in minutes so that you'll be able to run the required 8 or 12 miles by the beginning of cycle 6.

You don't need to increase your long runs any farther than 8 or 12 miles, but you can top out at 10 miles for 15-K training and 14 for the half-marathon. Don't go any farther. So, for example, if you are training for a 15-K and you cover 10 miles in your long run of 1 hour 50 minutes in cycle 5, keep your long run there for cycle 6.

Your workouts for day 7 will also increase in length but not to the same degree as the long run. Keep these workouts at a 51 RBE. You have the option of doing all of your workouts at 51 as in your base training or including the quality workouts given in each cycle.

SCHEDULE **A**:
15–K to Half–Marathon
Cycle 1 (weeks 1 and 2)

DAY	WEEKDAY	WORKOUT	RUN (TOTAL MINUTES @ 51 RBE)	QUALITY WORKOUTS (MINUTES @ RBE) OPTIONAL	
1	Sunday	long run	70		
2	Monday	easy	0		
3	Tuesday	moderate	15–20		
4	Wednesday	long intervals	25–30	10 min @ 51	
				2 min @ 31 2 min @ 51	run 3 times
				5–10 min @ 51	
5	Thursday	easy	0		
6	Friday	moderate	15–20		
7	Saturday	longer	35		
8	Sunday	easy	0		
9	Monday	moderate	15–20		
10	Tuesday	long intervals	25–30	10 min @ 51 3 min @ 31 3 min @ 51 3 min @ 31 10 min @ 51	
11	Wednesday	easy	0		
12	Thursday	moderate	15–20		
13	Friday	short intervals	15–20	5 min @ 51	
				1 min @ 32 1 min @ 51	run 5 times
				5 min @ 51	
14	Saturday	zero	0		

SCHEDULE **A**:
15-K to Half-Marathon
Cycle 2 (weeks 3 and 4)

DAY	WEEKDAY	WORKOUT	RUN (TOTAL MINUTES @ 51 RBE)	QUALITY WORKOUTS (MINUTES @ RBE) OPTIONAL	
1	Sunday	long run	80		
2	Monday	easy	0		
3	Tuesday	moderate	15–20		
4	Wednesday	long intervals	25–30	10 min @ 51	
				2 min @ 31 2 min @ 51	run 3 times
				5–10 min @ 51	
5	Thursday	easy	0		
6	Friday	moderate	15–20		
7	Saturday	longer	45		
8	Sunday	easy	0		
9	Monday	moderate	15–20		
10	Tuesday	long intervals	25–30	10 min @ 51 3 min @ 31 3 min @ 51 3 min @ 31 10 min @ 51	
11	Wednesday	easy	0		
12	Thursday	moderate	15–20		
13	Friday	short intervals	15–20	5 min @ 51	
				1 min @ 32 1 min @ 51	run 5 times
				5 min @ 51	
14	Saturday	zero	0		

SCHEDULE **A:**
15–K to Half–Marathon
Cycle 3 (weeks 5 and 6)

DAY	WEEKDAY	WORKOUT	RUN (TOTAL MINUTES @ 51 RBE)	QUALITY WORKOUTS (MINUTES @ RBE) OPTIONAL	
1	Sunday	long run	90		
2	Monday	easy	0		
3	Tuesday	moderate	15–20		
4	Wednesday	long intervals	25–30	10 min. @ 51	
				2 min @ 31 2 min @ 51	run 3 times
				5–10 min @ 51	
5	Thursday	easy	0		
6	Friday	moderate	15–20		
7	Saturday	longer	55		
8	Sunday	easy	0		
9	Monday	moderate	15–20		
10	Tuesday	long intervals	25–30	10 min @ 51 3 min @ 32 3 min @ 51 3 min @ 32 10 min @ 51	
11	Wednesday	easy	0		
12	Thursday	moderate	15–20		
13	Friday	short intervals	15–20	5 min @ 51 run	
				30 sec @ 32 1 min @ 51	5 to 7 times
				5 min @ 51	
14	Saturday	zero	0		

SCHEDULE A:
15-K to Half-Marathon
Cycle 4 (weeks 7 and 8)

DAY	WEEKDAY	WORKOUT	RUN (TOTAL MINUTES @ 51 RBE)	QUALITY WORKOUTS (MINUTES @ RBE) OPTIONAL
1	Sunday	long run	1 hr 40 min	
2	Monday	easy	0	
3	Tuesday	moderate	15–20	
4	Wednesday	long intervals	25–30	10 min @ 51 1 min @ 32 1 min @ 51 2 min @ 32 2 min @ 51 3 min @ 31 5–10 min @ 51
5	Thursday	easy	0	
6	Friday	moderate	15–20	
7	Saturday	longer	65	
8	Sunday	easy	0	
9	Monday	moderate	15–20	
10	Tuesday	long intervals	25–30	10 min @ 51 3 min @ 32 2 min @ 51 3 min @ 32 10 min @ 51
11	Wednesday	easy	0	
12	Thursday	moderate	15–20	
13	Friday	short intervals	15–20	5 min @ 51 30 sec @ 33 1 min @ 51 run 1 min @ 2 or 3 33 times 1 min @ 51 times 5 min @ 51
14	Saturday	zero	0	

SCHEDULE **A**:
15-K to Half-Marathon
Cycle 5 (weeks 9 and 10)

DAY	WEEKDAY	WORKOUT	RUN (TOTAL MINUTES @ 51 RBE)	QUALITY WORKOUTS (MINUTES @ RBE) OPTIONAL	
1	Sunday	long run	1 hr 50 min		
2	Monday	easy	0		
3	Tuesday	moderate	15–20		
4	Wednesday	long intervals	25–30	10 min @ 51 1 min @ 32 1 min @ 51 2 min @ 32 2 min @ 51 3 min @ 31 5–10 min @ 51	
5	Thursday	easy	0		
6	Friday	moderate	15–20		
7	Saturday	easy	75		
8	Sunday	longer	0		
9	Monday	moderate	15–20		
10	Tuesday	long intervals	25–30	10 min @ 51 3 min @ 32 2 min @ 51 3 min @ 32 10 min @ 51	
11	Wednesday	easy	0		
12	Thursday	moderate	15–20		
13	Friday	short intervals	15–20	5 min @ 51	
				30 sec @ 33 1 min @ 51 1 min @ 33 1 min @ 51	run 2 or 3 times
				5 min @ 51	
14	Saturday	zero	0		

SCHEDULE A:
15-K to Half-Marathon
Cycle 6 (weeks 11 and 12)

DAY	WEEKDAY	WORKOUT	RUN (TOTAL MINUTES @ 51 RBE)	QUALITY WORKOUTS (MINUTES @ RBE) OPTIONAL
1	Sunday	long run	2 hrs	
2	Monday	easy	0	
3	Tuesday	moderate	15–20	
4	Wednesday	long intervals	25–30	10 min @ 51 1 min @ 32 1 min @ 51 2 min @ 32 2 min @ 51 3 min @ 31 5–10 min @ 51
5	Thursday	easy	0	
6	Friday	moderate	15–20	
7	Saturday	longer	50	
8	Sunday	easy	0	
9	Monday	moderate	15–20	
10	Tuesday	long intervals	25–30	10 min @ 51 3 min @ 32 2 min @ 51 3 min @ 32 10 min @ 51
11	Wednesday	easy	0	
12	Thursday	moderate	15–20	
13	Friday	short intervals	15–20	5 min @ 51 [30 sec @ 33 / 1 min @ 51 / 1 min @ 33 / 1 min @ 51] run 2 or 3 times 5 min @ 51
14	Saturday	zero	0	

SCHEDULE **A**:
Taper and Recovery
(days leading up to and following the race)

DAY	WEEKDAY	RUN (TOTAL MINUTES @ 51 RBE)	QUALITY WORKOUTS (MINUTES @ RBE) OPTIONAL	
1	Sunday	25–30		
2	Monday	0		
3	Tuesday	15–20		
4	Wednesday	15	5 min @ 51	
			1 min @ 31 1 min @ 51	run 2 or 3 times
			5 min @ 51	
5	Thursday	0		
6	Friday	0–10		
7	Saturday	10–15		
8	Sunday	**RACE**	5 min @ 51 **RACE** 5 min @ 51 or walk	
9	Monday	0		
10	Tuesday	0		
11	Wednesday	15–20	15–20 min @ 51	
12	Thursday	0		
13	Friday	15	5 min @ 51	
			30 sec @ 52 1 min @ 51	run 2 or 3 times
			5 min @ 51	
14	Saturday	0		

Schedule A: Marathon

This bare minimum schedule will gradually enhance your endurance enough to cover the marathon distance. Still, it requires nine cycles of training—18 weeks—plus a taper. The key workouts are the long run on day 1 and the moderately long run on day 7. Be sure to keep your rhythmic breathing effort at 51 for these workouts, and keep in mind that they are essential to your success in the marathon (you really don't want to miss them). Quality workouts are included beginning with cycle 4 (weeks 7 and 8), but these are optional; you can choose to simply run the distance (minutes) scheduled at 51.

SCHEDULE **A**: Marathon
Cycle 1 (weeks 1 and 2)

DAY	WEEKDAY	WORKOUT	RUN (TOTAL MINUTES @ 51 RBE)	QUALITY WORKOUTS (MINUTES @ RBE) NONE
1	Sunday	long run	60	
2	Monday	easy	0	
3	Tuesday	moderate	15–20	
4	Wednesday	long intervals	25–30	
5	Thursday	easy	0	
6	Friday	moderate	15–20	
7	Saturday	longer	40	
8	Sunday	easy	0	
9	Monday	moderate	15–20	
10	Tuesday	long intervals	25–30	
11	Wednesday	easy	0	
12	Thursday	moderate	15–20	
13	Friday	short intervals	15–20	
14	Saturday	zero	0	

SCHEDULE **A**: Marathon
Cycle 2 (weeks 3 and 4)

DAY	WEEKDAY	WORKOUT	RUN (TOTAL MINUTES @ 51 RBE)	QUALITY WORKOUTS (MINUTES @ RBE) NONE
1	Sunday	long run	70	
2	Monday	easy	0	
3	Tuesday	moderate	15–20	
4	Wednesday	long intervals	25–30	
5	Thursday	easy	0	
6	Friday	moderate	15–20	
7	Saturday	longer	50	
8	Sunday	easy	0	
9	Monday	moderate	15–20	
10	Tuesday	long intervals	25–30	
11	Wednesday	easy	0	
12	Thursday	moderate	15–20	
13	Friday	short intervals	15–20	
14	Saturday	zero	0	

SCHEDULE **A**: Marathon
Cycle 3 (weeks 5 and 6)

DAY	WEEKDAY	WORKOUT	RUN (TOTAL MINUTES @ 51 RBE)	QUALITY WORKOUTS (MINUTES @ RBE) NONE
1	Sunday	long run	80	
2	Monday	easy	0	
3	Tuesday	moderate	15–20	
4	Wednesday	long intervals	25–30	
5	Thursday	easy	0	
6	Friday	moderate	15–20	
7	Saturday	longer	60	
8	Sunday	easy	0	
9	Monday	moderate	15–20	
10	Tuesday	long intervals	25–30	
11	Wednesday	easy	0	
12	Thursday	moderate	15–20	
13	Friday	short intervals	15–20	
14	Saturday	zero	0	

SCHEDULE **A**: Marathon
Cycle 4 (weeks 7 and 8)

DAY	WEEKDAY	WORKOUT	RUN (TOTAL MINUTES @ 51 RBE)	QUALITY WORKOUTS (MINUTES @ RBE) OPTIONAL	
1	Sunday	long run	1 hr 35 min		
2	Monday	easy	0		
3	Tuesday	moderate	15–20		
4	Wednesday	long intervals	25–30	10 min @ 51	
				2 min @ 31 2 min @ 51	run 3 times
				5–10 min @ 51	
5	Thursday	easy	0		
6	Friday	moderate	15–20		
7	Saturday	longer	70		
8	Sunday	easy	0		
9	Monday	moderate	15–20		
10	Tuesday	long intervals	25–30	10 min @ 51 3 min @ 31 3 min @ 51 3 min @ 31 10 min @ 51	
11	Wednesday	easy	0		
12	Thursday	moderate	15–20		
13	Friday	short intervals	15–20	5 min @ 51	
				1 min @ 32 1 min @ 51	run 5 times
				5 min @ 51	
14	Saturday	zero	0		

SCHEDULE **A**: Marathon
Cycle 5 (weeks 9 and 10)

DAY	WEEKDAY	WORKOUT	RUN (TOTAL MINUTES @ 51 RBE)	QUALITY WORKOUTS (MINUTES @ RBE) OPTIONAL	
1	Sunday	long run	1 hr 50 min		
2	Monday	easy	0		
3	Tuesday	moderate	15–20		
4	Wednesday	long intervals	25–30	10 min @ 51	
				2 min @ 31 2 min @ 51	run 3 times
				5–10 min @ 51	
5	Thursday	easy	0		
6	Friday	moderate	15–20		
7	Saturday	longer	80		
8	Sunday	easy	0		
9	Monday	moderate	15–20		
10	Tuesday	long intervals	25–30	10 min @ 51 3 min @ 31 3 min @ 51 3 min @ 31 10 min @ 51	
11	Wednesday	easy	0		
12	Thursday	moderate	15–20		
13	Friday	short intervals	15–20	5 min @ 51	
				1 min @ 32 1 min @ 51	run 5 times
				5 min @ 51	
14	Saturday	zero	0		

SCHEDULE **A**: Marathon
Cycle 6 (weeks 11 and 12)

DAY	WEEKDAY	WORKOUT	RUN (TOTAL MINUTES @ RBE 51)	QUALITY WORKOUTS (MINUTES @ RBE) OPTIONAL	
1	Sunday	long run	2 hrs 5 min		
2	Monday	easy	0		
3	Tuesday	moderate	15–20		
4	Wednesday	long intervals	25–30	10 min @ 51	
				2 min @ 31 2 min @ 51	run 3 times
				5–10 min @ 51	
5	Thursday	easy	0		
6	Friday	moderate	15–20		
7	Saturday	longer	1 hr 40 min		
8	Sunday	easy	0		
9	Monday	moderate	15–20		
10	Tuesday	long intervals	25–30	10 min @ 51 3 min @ 32 3 min @ 51 3 min @ 32 10 min @ 51	
11	Wednesday	easy	0		
12	Thursday	moderate	15–20		
13	Friday	short intervals	15–20	5 min @ 51 run	
				30 sec @ 32 1 min @ 51	5 to 7 times
				5 min @ 51	
14	Saturday	zero	0		

SCHEDULE **A**: Marathon
Cycle 7 (weeks 13 and 14)

DAY	WEEKDAY	WORKOUT	RUN (TOTAL MINUTES @ RBE 51)	QUALITY WORKOUTS (MINUTES @ RBE) OPTIONAL	
1	Sunday	long run	2 hrs 20 min		
2	Monday	easy	0		
3	Tuesday	moderate	15–20		
4	Wednesday	long intervals	25–30	10 min @ 51	
				2 min @ 31 2 min @ 51	run 3 times
				5–10 min @ 51	
5	Thursday	easy	0		
6	Friday	moderate	15–20		
7	Saturday	longer	1 hr 45 min		
8	Sunday	easy	0		
9	Monday	moderate	15–20		
10	Tuesday	long intervals	25–30	10 min @ 51 3 min @ 32 3 min @ 51 3 min @ 32 10 min @ 51	
11	Wednesday	easy	0		
12	Thursday	moderate	15–20		
13	Friday	short intervals	15–20	5 min @ 51	
				30 sec @ 32 1 min @ 51	run 5 to 7 times
				5 min @ 51	
14	Saturday	zero	0		

SCHEDULE A: Marathon
Cycle 8 (weeks 15 and 16)

DAY	WEEKDAY	WORKOUT	RUN (TOTAL MINUTES @ 51 RBE)	QUALITY WORKOUTS (MINUTES @ RBE) OPTIONAL
1	Sunday	long run	2 hr 40 min	
2	Monday	easy	0	
3	Tuesday	moderate	15–20	
4	Wednesday	long intervals	25–30	10 min @ 51 1 min @ 32 1 min @ 51 2 min @ 32 2 min @ 51 3 min @ 31 5–10 min @ 51
5	Thursday	easy	0	
6	Friday	moderate	15–20	
7	Saturday	longer	1 hr 45 min	
8	Sunday	easy	0	
9	Monday	moderate	15–20	
10	Tuesday	long intervals	25–30	10 min @ 51 3 min @ 32 2 min @ 51 3 min @ 32 10 min @ 51
11	Wednesday	easy	0	
12	Thursday	moderate	15–20	
13	Friday	short intervals	15–20	5 min @ 51 [30 sec @ 33 / 1 min @ 51 / 1 min @ 33 / 1 min @ 51] run 2 or 3 times 5 min @ 51
14	Saturday	zero	0	

SCHEDULE **A**: Marathon
Cycle 9 (weeks 17 and 18)

DAY	WEEKDAY	WORKOUT	RUN (TOTAL MINUTES @ 51 RBE)	QUALITY WORKOUTS (MINUTES @ RBE) OPTIONAL
1	Sunday	long run	3 hrs	
2	Monday	easy	0	
3	Tuesday	moderate	15–20	
4	Wednesday	long intervals	25–30	10 min @ 51 1 min @ 32 1 min @ 51 2 min @ 32 2 min @ 51 3 min @ 31 5–10 min @ 51
5	Thursday	easy	0	
6	Friday	moderate	15–20	
7	Saturday	longer	1 hr 45 min	
8	Sunday	easy	0	
9	Monday	moderate	15–20	
10	Tuesday	long intervals	25–30	10 min @ 51 3 min @ 32 2 min @ 51 3 min @ 32 10 min @ 51
11	Wednesday	easy	0	
12	Thursday	moderate	15–20	
13	Friday	short intervals	15–20	5 min @ 51 30 sec @ 33 / 1 min @ 51 / 1 min @ 33 / 1 min @ 51 — run 2 or 3 times 5 min @ 51
14	Saturday	zero	0	

SCHEDULE **A**: Marathon Taper and Recovery
(days leading up to and following the race)

DAY	WEEKDAY	RUN (TOTAL MINUTES @ 51 RBE)	QUALITY WORKOUTS (MINUTES @ RBE) OPTIONAL	
1	Sunday	60		
2	Monday	0		
3	Tuesday	15–20		
4	Wednesday	15	5 min @ 51	
			1 min @ 31 1 min @ 51	run 2 or 3 times
			5 min @ 51	
5	Thursday	0		
6	Friday	0–10		
7	Saturday	20		
8	Sunday	**RACE**	5 min @ 51 **RACE** 5 min @ 51 or walk	
9	Monday	0		
10	Tuesday	0		
11	Wednesday	15–20	15–20 min @ 51	
12	Thursday	0		
13	Friday	15	5 min @ 51	
			30 sec @ 52 1 min @ 51	run 2 or 3 times
			5 min @ 51	
14	Saturday	0		

Schedule B: 15-K to Marathon

Running the B level of base training has elevated your fitness and put you in excellent shape to train and race a 15-K, 10-miler, or half-marathon. Now it's time to add quality workouts to the mix. Your long runs lengthen, but you don't need to cover any more than 10 to 12 miles in training for the 15-K and 15 to 18 miles for the half, regardless of the times shown in the schedule. Six cycles—12 weeks—will get you ready for these longer distances. If the marathon is your goal, add the 6 weeks of training in the marathon extension.

SCHEDULE **B**:
15-K to Marathon
Cycle 1 (weeks 1 and 2)

DAY	WEEKDAY	WORKOUT	RUN (DISTANCE @ RBE)		
1	Sunday	long run	90 min @ 51		
2	Monday	easy	0–20 min @ 51		
3	Tuesday	moderate	30–40 min @ 51		
4	Wednesday	long intervals	10–15 min @ 51		
			2 min @ 31 2 min @ 51 4 min @ 31 2 min @ 51 6 min @ 31 3 min @ 51	run 2 times	
			10–15 min @ 51		
5	Thursday	easy	0–20 min @ 51		
6	Friday	moderate	30–40 min @ 51		
7	Saturday	tempo	10–15 min @ 51 10 min @ 52 2 min @ 51 10 min @ 52 10–15 min @ 51		
8	Sunday	easy	0–20 min @ 51		
9	Monday	moderate	30–40 min @ 51		
10	Tuesday	long intervals	10–15 min @ 51		
			3 min @ 31 3 min @ 51	run 3 to 4 times	
			10–15 min @ 51		
11	Wednesday	easy	0–20 min @ 51		
12	Thursday	moderate	30–40 min @ 51		
13	Friday	short intervals	10 min @ 51		
			1 min @ 31 1 min @ 51	run 8 to 10 times	
			10 min @ 51		
14	Saturday	zero	0		

SCHEDULE **B**:
15-K to Marathon
Cycle 2 (weeks 3 and 4)

DAY	WEEKDAY	WORKOUT	RUN (DISTANCE @ RBE)	
1	Sunday	long run	1 hr 45 min @ 51	
2	Monday	easy	0–20 min @ 51	
3	Tuesday	moderate	30–40 min @ 51	
4	Wednesday	long intervals	10–15 min @ 51	
			4 min @ 31 2 min @ 51	2 times
			6 min @ 31 3 min @ 51	1 time
			4 min @ 31 2 min @ 51	2 times
			10–15 min @ 51	
5	Thursday	easy	0–20 min @ 51	
6	Friday	moderate	30–40 min @ 51	
7	Saturday	tempo	10–15 min @ 51 15 min @ 52 5 min @ 51 5 min @ 52 10–15 min @ 51	
8	Sunday	easy	0–20 min @ 51	
9	Monday	moderate	30–40 min @ 51	
10	Tuesday	long intervals	10–15 min @ 51	
			3 min @ 31 2 min @ 51 1.5 min @ 31 1 min @ 51	run 3 to 4 times
			10–15 min @ 51	
11	Wednesday	easy	0–20 min @ 51	
12	Thursday	moderate	30–40 min @ 51	
13	Friday	short intervals	10 min @ 51	
			1 min @ 31 1 min @ 51	run 8 to 10 times
			10 min @ 51	
14	Saturday	zero	0	

SCHEDULE **B**:
15-K to Marathon
Cycles 3, 4, 5 (weeks 5 through 10)

DAY	WEEKDAY	WORKOUT	RUN (DISTANCE @ RBE)	
1	Sunday	long run	For 15-K: 2 hrs @ 51 For half-marathon: 2 hrs 15 min @ 51 For marathon: 2½ hrs @ 51	
2	Monday	easy	0–20 min @ 51	
3	Tuesday	moderate	30–40 min @ 51	
4	Wednesday	long intervals	10–15 min @ 51	
			6 min @ 31 3 min @ 51	run 3 or 4 times
			10–15 min @ 51	
5	Thursday	easy	0–20 min @ 51	
6	Friday	moderate	30–40 min @ 51	
7	Saturday	tempo	10–15 min @ 51 20 min @ 52 10–15 min @ 51 Run on course similar to 15-K or half-marathon course	
8	Sunday	easy	0–20 min @ 51	
9	Monday	moderate	30–40 min @ 51	
10	Tuesday	long intervals	10–15 min @ 51	
			3 min @ 31 2 min @ 51 1.5 min @ 31 1 min @ 51	run 3 or 4 times
			10–15 min @ 51 OR hill workout, see page 180	
11	Wednesday	easy	0–20 min @ 51	
12	Thursday	moderate	30–40 min @ 51	
13	Friday	short intervals	10 min @ 51	
			30 sec @ 32 1 min @ 51 1 min @ 32 1 min @ 51 1.5 min @ 32 4 min @ 51	run 3 or 4 times
			10 min @ 51	
14	Saturday	zero	0	

SCHEDULE **B**:
15-K to Marathon
Cycle 6 (weeks 11 and 12)

DAY	WEEKDAY	WORKOUT	RUN (DISTANCE @ RBE)	
1	Sunday	long run	2 hrs @ 51	
2	Monday	easy	0–20 min @ 51	
3	Tuesday	moderate	30–40 min @ 51	
4	Wednesday	long intervals	10–15 min @ 51	
			6 min @ 31 3 min @ 51 4 min @ 31 2 min @ 51 2 min @ 31 1 min @ 51 1 min @ 31 1 min @ 51	
			10–15 min @ 51	
5	Thursday	easy	0–20 min @ 51	
6	Friday	moderate	30–40 min @ 51	
7	Saturday	tempo	10–15 min @ 51 20 min @ 52 10 min @ 51	
8	Sunday	easy	0–20 min @ 51	
9	Monday	moderate	30–40 min @ 51	
10	Tuesday	long intervals	10–15 min @ 51	
			3 min @ 32 3 min @ 51 2 min @ 31 2 min @ 51 1 min @ 31 1 min @ 51	run 2 or 3 times
			10–15 min @ 51	
11	Wednesday	easy	0–20 min @ 51	
12	Thursday	moderate	30–40 min @ 51	
13	Friday	short intervals	10 min @ 51	
			30 sec @ 32 30 sec @ 51	run 10 to 15 times
			10 min @ 51	
14	Saturday	zero	0	

SCHEDULE **B**:
Taper
(days leading up to and following the race)

DAY	WEEKDAY	RUN (DISTANCE @ RBE)		
1	Sunday	40–50 min @ 51		
2	Monday	0		
3	Tuesday	20–30 min @ 51		
4	Wednesday	10 min @ 51		
		1.5 min @ 31 1.5 min @ 51	run 3 to 5 times	
		10 min @ 51		
5	Thursday	0–15 min @ 51		
6	Friday	0		
7	Saturday	15–20 min @ 51		
8	Sunday	5–10 min @ 51 or walk **RACE:** 15-K to half-marathon Walk 5–10 min		
9	Monday	0–20 min @ 51		
10	Tuesday	20–30 min @ 51		
11	Wednesday	0–20 min @ 51		
12	Thursday	30–40 min @ 51		
13	Friday	30–40 min @ 51		
14	Saturday	0		

SCHEDULE **B**:
Marathon Extension
Cycle 7 (weeks 13 and 14)

DAY	WEEKDAY	WORKOUT	RUN (DISTANCE @ RBE)	
1	Sunday	long run	60–90 min @ 51	
2	Monday	easy	0–20 min @ 51	
3	Tuesday	moderate	30–40 min @ 51	
4	Wednesday	long intervals	10–15 min @ 51	
			4 min @ 31 2 min @ 51 6 min @ 31 2 min @ 51 4 min @ 31 2 min @ 51	run 1 or 2 times
			10–15 min @ 51	
5	Thursday	easy	0–20 min @ 51	
6	Friday	moderate	30–40 min @ 51	
7	Saturday	tempo	10–15 min @ 51 20 min @ 52 2 min @ 51 10 min @ 52 10–15 min @ 51 Run on course similar to marathon course	
8	Sunday	easy	0–20 min @ 51	
9	Monday	moderate	30–40 min @ 51	
10	Tuesday	long intervals	10–15 min @ 51	
			3 min @ 31 3 min @ 51	run 4 or 5 times
			10–15 min @ 51	
11	Wednesday	easy	0–20 min @ 51	
12	Thursday	moderate	30–40 min @ 51	
13	Friday	short intervals	10 min @ 51	
			1 min @ 31 1 min @ 51	run 5 to 10 times
			10 min @ 51	
14	Saturday	zero	0	

SCHEDULE **B**:
Marathon Extension
Cycle 8 (weeks 15 and 16)

DAY	WEEKDAY	WORKOUT	RUN (DISTANCE @ RBE)	
1	Sunday	long run	2–2½ hrs @ 51	
2	Monday	easy	0–20 min @ 51	
3	Tuesday	moderate	30–40 min @ 51	
4	Wednesday	long intervals	10–15 min @ 51 4 min @ 31 2 min @ 51 6 min @ 31	
			3 min @ 51 8 min @ 31	run 1 or 2 times
			10–15 min @ 51	
5	Thursday	easy	0–20 min @ 51	
6	Friday	moderate	30–40 min @ 51	
7	Saturday	tempo	10–15 min @ 51 30–35 min @ 52 10–15 min @ 51	
8	Sunday	easy	0–20 min @ 51	
9	Monday	moderate	30–40 min @ 51	
10	Tuesday	long intervals	10–15 min @ 51	
			4 min @ 31 3 min @ 51	run 3 to 5 times
			10–15 min @ 51	
11	Wednesday	easy	0–20 min @ 51	
12	Thursday	moderate	30–40 min @ 51	
13	Friday	short intervals	10 min @ 51	
			1 min @ 31 1 min @ 51	run 5 to 10 times
			10 min @ 51	
14	Saturday	zero	0	

SCHEDULE **B**:
Marathon Extension
Cycle 9 (weeks 17 and 18)

DAY	WEEKDAY	WORKOUT	RUN (DISTANCE @ RBE)	
1	Sunday	long run	2½–3 hrs @ 51	
2	Monday	easy	0–20 min @ 51	
3	Tuesday	moderate	30–40 min @ 51	
4	Wednesday	long intervals	10–15 min @ 51	
			6 min @ 31 3 min @ 51 8 min @ 31	run 2 times
			10 min @ 51	
5	Thursday	easy	0–20 min @ 51	
6	Friday	moderate	30–40 min @ 51	
7	Saturday	tempo	10–15 min @ 51 20 min @ 52 10 min @ 51	
8	Sunday	easy	0–20 min @ 51	
9	Monday	moderate	30–40 min @ 51	
10	Tuesday	long intervals	10–15 min @ 51	
			2 min @ 31 2 min @ 51 3 min @ 31 3 min @ 51 2 min @ 31 2 min @ 51	run 2 times
			10–15 min @ 51	
11	Wednesday	easy	0–20 min	
12	Thursday	moderate	30–40 min	
13	Friday	short intervals	10 min @ 51	
			1 min @ 31 1 min @ 51	run 5 to 10 times
			10 min @ 51	
14	Saturday	zero	0	

SCHEDULE **B**:
Marathon Taper
(days leading up to and following the race)

DAY	WEEKDAY	RUN (DISTANCE @ RBE)		
1	Sunday	40–50 min @ 51		
2	Monday	0		
3	Tuesday	20–30 min @ 51		
4	Wednesday	10 min @ 51		
		1.5 min @ 31 1.5 min @ 51	run 3 to 5 times	
		10 min @ 51		
5	Thursday	0–15 min @ 51		
6	Friday	0		
7	Saturday	15–20 min @ 51		
8	Sunday	Walk 10–15 min **RACE:** Marathon Walk 10–15 min		
9	Monday	0–20 min @ 51		
10	Tuesday	0–20 min @ 51		
11	Wednesday	0–20 min @ 51		
12	Thursday	30–40 min @ 51		
13	Friday	10–20 min @ 51		
14	Saturday	0		

Schedules C and D: 15-K through the Marathon

You are serious. You dedicate a large part of your day to your training. And if your long runs cover close to 18 miles, these schedules do not require you to spend any more time running. What does change is the composition of your quality workouts. But before you read one sentence more, take another look at the 14-day training schedule on pages 88–91. You'll see a range in running distances for each day. You have a choice, and you need to make a smart one. If you're feeling great and have noticed improved fitness as you progress from cycle to cycle, go ahead and run at the top end of the range. If you're a bit worn out and find that you don't look forward to each day's run, opt for a shorter run. And if, after 5 to 10 minutes of running, you just don't have it that day, stop and walk home. My rule is this: When in doubt, don't. Another way to check your body's level of fatigue is by taking your pulse every morning and tracking it in your training log. If you notice your heart rate rising above what is typical for you, it's a good sign that you're overdoing it. (See page 173 for more details on morning heart rate and what it means for you.)

A few additional key points: Though the distances for your long runs are given in hours and minutes, set a goal of covering 18 miles. Running those 18 miles on a flat course will, of course, take less time than if you set out over the hills. Finding a long run that travels a similar path of hills and flats to your goal marathon can significantly enhance your readiness for race day. Remember to run all of your workouts at the recommended rhythmic breathing effort. If you're feeling frisky, rein it in—running too fast for any given workout will defeat its purpose.

SCHEDULE C:
15-K through the Marathon
Cycle 1 (weeks 1 and 2)

DAY	WEEKDAY	WORKOUT	RUN (DISTANCE @ RBE)		
1	Sunday	long run	1½–2 hrs @ 51		
2	Monday	easy	30–40 min @ 51		
3	Tuesday	moderate	40–60 min @ 51		
4	Wednesday	long intervals	15–20 min @ 51		
			4 min @ 31 2 min @ 51 6 min @ 31 2 min @ 51	run 2 or 3 times	
			15–20 min @ 51		
5	Thursday	easy	0–30 min @ 51		
6	Friday	moderate	40–60 min @ 51		
7	Saturday	tempo	15–20 min @ 51 10 min @ 52 2 min @ 51 10 min @ 52 2 min @ 51 5 min @ 52 15–20 min @ 51		
8	Sunday	easy	0–30 min @ 51		
9	Monday	moderate	40–60 min @ 51		
10	Tuesday	long intervals	15–20 min @ 51		
			3 min @ 31 3 min @ 51	run 5 to 7 times	
			15–20 min @ 51		
11	Wednesday	easy	0–30 min @ 51		
12	Thursday	moderate	40–60 min @ 51		
13	Friday	short intervals	10 min @ 51		
			1 min @ 32 1 min @ 51	run 10 to 15 times	
			10 min @ 51		
14	Saturday	zero	0		

SCHEDULE C:
15–K through the Marathon
Cycle 2 (weeks 3 and 4)

DAY	WEEKDAY	WORKOUT	RUN (DISTANCE @ RBE)	
1	Sunday	long run	1½–2 hrs @ 51	
2	Monday	easy	30–40 min @ 51	
3	Tuesday	moderate	40–60 min @ 51	
4	Wednesday	long intervals	15–20 min @ 51	
			4 min @ 31 2 min @ 51	2 times
			6 min @ 31 3 min @ 51	2 times
			4 min @ 31 2 min @ 51	2 times
			15–20 min @ 51	
5	Thursday	easy	0–30 min @ 51	
6	Friday	moderate	40–60 min @ 51	
7	Saturday	tempo	15–20 min @ 51 15 min @ 52 2 min @ 51 15 min @ 52 15–20 min @ 51	
8	Sunday	easy	0–30 min @ 51	
9	Monday	moderate	40–60 min @ 51	
10	Tuesday	long intervals	15–20 min @ 51	
			3 min @ 31 3 min @ 51 4 min @ 31 3 min @ 51	run 2 or 3 times
			15–20 min @ 51	
11	Wednesday	easy	0–30 min @ 51	
12	Thursday	moderate	40–60 min @ 51	
13	Friday	short intervals	10 min @ 51	
			1 min @ 32 1 min @ 51	run 10 to 15 times
			10 min @ 51	
14	Saturday	zero	0	

SCHEDULE **C:**
15-K through the Marathon
Cycles 3, 4, 5 (weeks 5 through 10)

DAY	WEEKDAY	WORKOUT	RUN (DISTANCE @ RBE)	
1	Sunday	long run	1¾–2 hrs @ 51	
2	Monday	easy	30–40 min @ 51	
3	Tuesday	moderate	40–60 min @ 51	
4	Wednesday	long intervals	15–20 min @ 51	
			6 min @ 31 3 min @ 51	run 3 to 5 times
			15–20 min @ 51	
5	Thursday	easy	0–30 min @ 51	
6	Friday	moderate	40–60 min @ 51	
7	Saturday	tempo	15–20 min @ 51 30 min @ 52 15–20 min @ 51 OR 5-K to 10-K race	
8	Sunday	easy	0–30 min @ 51	
9	Monday	moderate	40–60 min @ 51	
10	Tuesday	long intervals	15–20 min @ 51	
			4 min @ 31 3 min @ 51	run 4 to 6 times
			15–20 min @ 51 OR hill workout, see page 177	
11	Wednesday	easy	0–30 min @ 51	
12	Thursday	moderate	40–60 min @ 51	
13	Friday	short intervals	10 min @ 51	
			30 sec @ 31 1 min @ 51 1 min @ 31 1 min @ 51 1.5 min @ 31 1 min @ 51	run 4 to 7 times
			10 min @ 51	
14	Saturday	zero	0	

SCHEDULE **C**:
15–K through the Marathon
Cycle 6 (weeks 11 and 12)

DAY	WEEKDAY	WORKOUT	RUN (DISTANCE @ RBE)	
1	Sunday	long run	90 min @ 51	
2	Monday	easy	30–40 min @ 51	
3	Tuesday	moderate	40–60 min @ 51	
4	Wednesday	long intervals	15–20 min @ 51	
			4 min @ 31 2 min @ 51	run 3 to 6 times
			15–20 min @ 51	
5	Thursday	easy	0–30 min @ 51	
6	Friday	moderate	40–60 min @ 51	
7	Saturday	tempo	15–20 min @ 51 20 min @ 31 15–20 min @ 51 OR 5-K race	
8	Sunday	easy	0–30 min @ 51	
9	Monday	moderate	40–60 min @ 51	
10	Tuesday	long intervals	10–15 min @ 51	
			2 min @ 31 2 min @ 51	run 4 to 8 times
			15–20 min @ 51	
11	Wednesday	easy	0–30 min @ 51	
12	Thursday	moderate	40–60 min @ 51	
13	Friday	short intervals	10 min @ 51	
			30 sec @ 32 30 sec @ 51	run 10 to 15 times
			10 min @ 51	
14	Saturday	zero	0	

SCHEDULE **C**: Taper
15-K to Half-Marathon
(days leading up to and following the race)

DAY	WEEKDAY	RUN (DISTANCE @ RBE)	
1	Sunday	60–80 min @ 51	
2	Monday	0	
3	Tuesday	30–40 min @ 51	
4	Wednesday	15–20 min @ 51	
		1.5 min @ 31 1.5 min @ 51	run 5 to 7 times
		10 min @ 51	
5	Thursday	15–20 min @ 51	
6	Friday	0	
7	Saturday	15–20 min @ 51	
8	Sunday	10–15 min @ 51 **RACE:** 15-K to half-marathon 10–15 min @ 51 or walk	
9	Monday	20–30 min @ 51	
10	Tuesday	30–40 min @ 51	
11	Wednesday	20–30 min @ 51	
12	Thursday	30–40 min @ 51	
13	Friday	30–40 min @ 51	
14	Saturday	0	

SCHEDULE **C**:
Marathon Extension
Cycle 7 (weeks 13 and 14)

DAY	WEEKDAY	WORKOUT	RUN (DISTANCE @ RBE)	
1	Sunday	long run	60–90 min @ 51	
2	Monday	easy	30–40 min @ 51	
3	Tuesday	moderate	40–60 min @ 51	
4	Wednesday	long intervals	15–20 min @ 51	
			1 min @ 31 1 min @ 51	run 6 to 8 times
			15–20 min @ 51	
5	Thursday	easy	0–30 min @ 51	
6	Friday	moderate	40–60 min @ 51	
7	Saturday	tempo	15–20 min @ 51 20 min @ 52 5 min @ 51 20 min @ 52 15–20 min @ 51 Run on course similar to marathon	
8	Sunday	easy	0–30 min @ 51	
9	Monday	moderate	40–60 min @ 51	
10	Tuesday	long intervals	15–20 min @ 51	
			3 min @ 31 3 min @ 51	run 5 to 7 times
			15–20 min @ 51	
11	Wednesday	easy	0–30 min @ 51	
12	Thursday	moderate	40–60 min @ 51	
13	Friday	short intervals	10 min @ 51	
			1 min @ 31 1 min @ 51	run 15 to 20 times
			10 min @ 51	
14	Saturday	zero	0	

SCHEDULE **C**:
Marathon Extension
Cycle 8 (weeks 15 and 16)

DAY	WEEKDAY	WORKOUT	RUN (DISTANCE @ RBE)		
1	Sunday	long run	2–2½ hrs @ 51		
2	Monday	easy	30–40 min @ 51		
3	Tuesday	moderate	40–60 min @ 51		
4	Wednesday	long intervals	15–20 min @ 51 20 min @ 52–31 8 min @ 51		
			1.5 min @ 31 1.5 min @ 51	run 6 to 8 times	
			15–20 min @ 51		
5	Thursday	easy	0–30 min @ 51		
6	Friday	moderate	40–60 min @ 51		
7	Saturday	tempo	15–20 min @ 51 30–40 min @ 52 15–20 min @ 51 Run on course similar to marathon		
8	Sunday	easy	0–30 min @ 51		
9	Monday	moderate	40–60 min @ 51		
10	Tuesday	long intervals	15–20 min @ 51		
			3 min @ 31 3 min @ 51	run 5 to 7 times	
			15–20 min @ 51		
11	Wednesday	easy	0–30 min @ 51		
12	Thursday	moderate	40–60 min @ 51		
13	Friday	short intervals	10 min @ 51		
			1 min @ 31 1 min @ 51	run 15 to 20 times	
			10 min @ 51		
14	Saturday	zero	0		

SCHEDULE **C**:
Marathon Extension
Cycle 9 (weeks 17 and 18)

DAY	WEEKDAY	WORKOUT	RUN (DISTANCE @ RBE)	
1	Sunday	long run	2½ hrs @ 51	
2	Monday	easy	30–40 min @ 51	
3	Tuesday	moderate	40–60 min @ 51	
4	Wednesday	long intervals	15–20 min @ 51	
			3 min @ 31 min @ 51 5 min @ 31 3 min @ 51 3 min @ 31 2 min @ 51	run 2 times
			15–20 min @ 51	
5	Thursday	easy	0–30 min @ 51	
6	Friday	moderate	40–60 min @ 51	
7	Saturday	tempo	15–20 min @ 51 20 min @ 31–32 15–20 min @ 51 OR 5-K race	
8	Sunday	easy	0–30 min @ 51	
9	Monday	moderate	40–60 min @ 51	
10	Tuesday	long intervals	15 min @ 51	
			6 min @ 31 4 min @ 51 5 min @ 31 3 min @ 51 3 min @ 31 2 min @ 51 1 min @ 31 1 min @ 51	run 1 or 2 times
			10–15 min @ 51	
11	Wednesday	easy	0–30 min @ 51	
12	Thursday	moderate	40–60 min @ 51	
13	Friday	short intervals	10 min @ 51	
			1 min @ 31 1 min @ 51	run 10 times
			10 min @ 51	
14	Saturday	zero	0	

SCHEDULE C:
Taper Marathon
(days leading up to and following the race)

DAY	WEEKDAY	RUN (DISTANCE @ RBE)		
1	Sunday	60 min @ 51		
2	Monday	0		
3	Tuesday	30–40 min @ 51		
4	Wednesday	10–15 min @ 51		
		1.5 min @ 31 1.5 min @ 51	run 6 times	
		10–15 min @ 51		
5	Thursday	15–20 min @ 51		
6	Friday	0		
7	Saturday	15–20 min @ 51		
8	Sunday	10 min @ 51 **RACE:** Marathon 10 min @ 51 or walk		
9	Monday	20–30 min @ 51		
10	Tuesday	0–20 min @ 51		
11	Wednesday	20–30 min @ 51		
12	Thursday	30–40 min @ 51		
13	Friday	10–20 min @ 51		
14	Saturday	0		

SCHEDULE **D:**
15–K through the Marathon
Cycle 1 (weeks 1 and 2)

DAY	WEEKDAY	WORKOUT	RUN (DISTANCE @ RBE)	
1	Sunday	long run	1½–2 hrs @ 51	
2	Monday	easy	30–40 min @ 51	
3	Tuesday	moderate	60–80 min @ 51	
4	Wednesday	long intervals	15–20 min @ 51	
			4 min @ 31 2 min @ 51 6 min @ 31 3 min @ 51 4 min @ 31 2 min @ 51	run 2 or 3 times
			15–20 min @ 51	
5	Thursday	easy	30–40 min @ 51	
6	Friday	moderate	60–80 min @ 51	
7	Saturday	tempo	15–20 min @ 51 10 min @ 52 2 min @ 51 10 min @ 52 2 min @ 51 5 min @ 52 15–20 min @ 51	
8	Sunday	easy	0–30 min @ 51	
9	Monday	moderate	60–80 min @ 51	
10	Tuesday	long intervals	15–20 min @ 51	
			3 min @ 31 3 min @ 51	run 7 or 8 times
			15–20 min @ 51	
11	Wednesday	easy	30 min @ 51	
12	Thursday	moderate	50–60 min @ 51	
13	Friday	short intervals	10 min @ 51	
			1 min @ 32 1 min @ 51	run 15 to 20 times
			10 min @ 51	
14	Saturday	zero	0	

SCHEDULE **D**:
15-K through the Marathon
Cycle 2 (weeks 3 and 4)

DAY	WEEKDAY	WORKOUT	RUN (DISTANCE @ RBE)		
1	Sunday	long run	1½–2 hrs @ 51		
2	Monday	easy	30–40 min @ 51		
3	Tuesday	moderate	60–80 min @ 51		
4	Wednesday	long intervals	15–20 min @ 51 20 min @ 52–31 8 min @ 51		
			1.5 min @ 31 1.5 min @ 51	run 8 to 10 times	
			15–20 min @ 51		
5	Thursday	easy	30–40 min @ 51		
6	Friday	moderate	60–80 min @ 51		
7	Saturday	tempo	15–20 min @ 51 15 min @ 52 2 min @ 51 15 min @ 52 15–20 min @ 51		
8	Sunday	easy	0–30 min @ 51		
9	Monday	moderate	60–80 min @ 51		
10	Tuesday	long intervals	15–20 min @ 51		
			4 min @ 31 2 min @ 51 2 min @ 31 1 min @ 51	run 4 to 6 times	
			15–20 min @ 51		
11	Wednesday	easy	30 min @ 51		
12	Thursday	moderate	50–60 min @ 51		
13	Friday	short intervals	10 min @ 51		
			1 min @ 32 1 min @ 51	run 15 to 20 times	
			10 min @ 51		
14	Saturday	zero	0		

SCHEDULE **D**:
15-K through the Marathon
Cycles 3 and 4 (weeks 5 through 8)

DAY	WEEKDAY	WORKOUT	RUN (DISTANCE @ RBE)	
1	Sunday	long run	2 hrs @ 51	
2	Monday	easy	30–40 min @ 51	
3	Tuesday	moderate	60–80 min @ 51	
4	Wednesday	long intervals	15–20 min @ 51	
			6 min @ 31 3 min @ 51	run 4 to 8 times
			15–20 min @ 51	
5	Thursday	easy	30–40 min @ 51	
6	Friday	moderate	60–80 min @ 51	
7	Saturday	tempo	15–20 min @ 51 30 min @ 52 15–20 min @ 51 OR 5-K to 10-K race	
8	Sunday	easy	0–30 min @ 51	
9	Monday	moderate	60–80 min @ 51	
10	Tuesday	long intervals	15–20 min @ 51	
			4 min @ 31 2 min @ 51 2 min @ 31 1 min @ 51	run 4 to 6 times
			15–20 min @ 51 OR long hill repeats, see page 179	
11	Wednesday	easy	30 min @ 51	
12	Thursday	moderate	50–60 min @ 51	
13	Friday	short intervals	10 min @ 51	
			30–45 sec uphill @ 32 jog downhill @ 51	run 8 to 12 times
			10 min @ 51	
14	Saturday	zero	0	

SCHEDULE **D**:
15–K through the Marathon
Cycle 5 (weeks 9 and 10)

DAY	WEEKDAY	WORKOUT	RUN (DISTANCE @ RBE)		
1	Sunday	long run	2–2½ hrs @ 51		
2	Monday	easy	30–40 min @ 51		
3	Tuesday	moderate	60–80 min @ 51		
4	Wednesday	long intervals	15–20 min @ 51 20 min @ 52–31 8 min @ 51		
			1.5 min @ 31 1.5 min @ 51	run 8 to 10 times	
			15–20 min @ 51		
5	Thursday	easy	30–40 min @ 51		
6	Friday	moderate	60–80 min @ 51		
7	Saturday	tempo	15–20 min @ 51 30 min @ 52 15–20 min @ 51		
8	Sunday	easy	0–30 min @ 51		
9	Monday	moderate	60–80 min @ 51		
10	Tuesday	long intervals	15–20 min @ 51 OR long hill repeats, see page 179		
11	Wednesday	easy	30 min @ 51		
12	Thursday	moderate	50–60 min @ 51		
13	Friday	short intervals	10 min @ 51		
			30 sec @ 31 30 sec @ 51	run 15 to 20 times	
			10 min @ 51		
14	Saturday	zero	0		

SCHEDULE **D**:
15-K through the Marathon
Cycle 6 (weeks 11 and 12)

DAY	WEEKDAY	WORKOUT	RUN (DISTANCE @ RBE)	
1	Sunday	long run	1½–2 hrs @ 51	
2	Monday	easy	30–40 min @ 51	
3	Tuesday	moderate	60–80 min @ 51	
4	Wednesday	long intervals	15–20 min @ 51	
			4 min @ 31 2 min @ 51	run 4 to 7 times
			15–20 min @ 51	
5	Thursday	easy	30–40 min @ 51	
6	Friday	moderate	60–80 min @ 51	
7	Saturday	tempo	15–20 min @ 51 20 min @ 31 15–20 min @ 51 OR 5-K race	
8	Sunday	easy	0–30 min @ 51	
9	Monday	moderate	60–80 min @ 51	
10	Tuesday	long intervals	10–15 min @ 51	
			2 min @ 31 2 min @ 51	run 5 to 7 times
			10–15 min @ 51	
11	Wednesday	easy	30 min @ 51	
12	Thursday	moderate	50–60 min @ 51	
13	Friday	short intervals	10 min @ 51	
			30 sec @ 31 30 sec @ 51	run 15 to 20 times
			10 min @ 51	
14	Saturday	zero	0	

SCHEDULE **D**: Taper
15-K through Half-Marathon
(days leading up to and following the race)

DAY	WEEKDAY	RUN (DISTANCE @ RBE)		
1	Sunday	60–80 min @ 51		
2	Monday	0–30 min @ 51		
3	Tuesday	40–50 min @ 51		
4	Wednesday	15–20 min @ 51		
		1.5 min @ 31 1.5 min @ 51	run 5 to 7 times	
		15–20 min @ 51		
5	Thursday	20–30 min @ 51		
6	Friday	0		
7	Saturday	20 min @ 51		
8	Sunday	15–20 min @ 51 **RACE:** 15-K to half-marathon 10–15 min @ 51 or walk		
9	Monday	20–40 min @ 51		
10	Tuesday	30–40 min @ 51		
11	Wednesday	20–30 min @ 51		
12	Thursday	30–40 min @ 51		
13	Friday	30–40 min @ 51		
14	Saturday	0		

SCHEDULE **D**:
Marathon Extension
Cycle 7 (weeks 13 and 14)

DAY	WEEKDAY	WORKOUT	RUN (DISTANCE @ RBE)	
1	Sunday	long run	1–1½ hrs @ 51	
2	Monday	easy	30–40 min @ 51	
3	Tuesday	moderate	60–80 min @ 51	
4	Wednesday	long intervals	15–20 min @ 51	
			1 min @ 31 1 min @ 51	run 8 to 10 times
			15–20 min @ 51	
5	Thursday	easy	30–40 min @ 51	
6	Friday	moderate	60–80 min @ 51	
7	Saturday	tempo	15–20 min @ 51 20 min @ 52 5 min @ 51 20 min @ 52 15–20 min @ 51	
8	Sunday	easy	0–30 min @ 51	
9	Monday	moderate	60–80 min @ 51	
10	Tuesday	long intervals	15–20 min @ 51	
			3 min @ 31 3 min @ 51	run 6 to 8 times
			15–20 min @ 51	
11	Wednesday	easy	30 min @ 51	
12	Thursday	moderate	50–60 min @ 51	
13	Friday	short intervals	10 min @ 51	
			1 min @ 31 1 min @ 51	run 15 to 20 times
			10 min @ 51	
14	Saturday	zero	0	

SCHEDULE **D**:
Marathon Extension
Cycle 8 (weeks 15 and 16)

DAY	WEEKDAY	WORKOUT	RUN (DISTANCE @ RBE)		
1	Sunday	long run	2½ hrs @ 51		
2	Monday	easy	30–40 min @ 51		
3	Tuesday	moderate	60–80 min @ 51		
4	Wednesday	long intervals	15–20 min @ 51 20 min @ 52–31 8 min @ 51		
			1.5 min @ 31 1.5 min @ 51	run 8 to 10 times	
			15–20 min @ 51		
5	Thursday	easy	30–40 min @ 51		
6	Friday	moderate	60–80 min @ 51		
7	Saturday	tempo	15–20 min @ 51 40 min @ 52 15–20 min @ 51		
8	Sunday	easy	0–30 min @ 51		
9	Monday	moderate	60–80 min @ 51		
10	Tuesday	long intervals	15–20 min @ 51		
			4 min @ 31 3 min @ 51	run 5 to 8 times	
			15–20 min @ 51		
11	Wednesday	easy	30 min @ 51		
12	Thursday	moderate	50–60 min @ 51		
13	Friday	short intervals	10 min @ 51		
			1 min @ 31 1 min @ 51	run 15 to 20 times	
			10 min @ 51		
14	Saturday	zero	0		

SCHEDULE **D**:
Marathon Extension
Cycle 9 (weeks 17 and 18)

DAY	WEEKDAY	WORKOUT	RUN (DISTANCE @ RBE)	
1	Sunday	long run	2½–3 hrs @ 51	
2	Monday	easy	30–40 min @ 51	
3	Tuesday	moderate	60–80 min @ 51	
4	Wednesday	long intervals	15–20 min @ 51	
			3 min @ 31 2 min @ 51 5 min @ 31 3 min @ 51 3 min @ 31 2 min @ 51	run 2 or 3 times
			15–20 min @ 51	
5	Thursday	easy	30–40 min @ 51	
6	Friday	moderate	60–80 min @ 51	
7	Saturday	tempo	15–20 min @ 51 20 min @ 31–32 15–20 min @ 51 OR 5-K race	
8	Sunday	easy	0–30 min @ 51	
9	Monday	moderate	60–80 min @ 51	
10	Tuesday	long intervals	15–20 min @ 51	
			6 min @ 31 4 min @ 51 5 min @ 31 3 min @ 51 3 min @ 31 2 min @ 51 1 min @ 31 1 min @ 51	run 2 times
			10–15 min @ 51	
11	Wednesday	easy	30 min @ 51	
12	Thursday	moderate	50–60 min @ 51	
13	Friday	short intervals	10 min @ 51	
			1 min @ 31 1 min @ 51	run 10 times
			10 min @ 51	
14	Saturday	zero	0	

SCHEDULE **D**:
Taper Marathon
(days leading up to and following the race)

DAY	WEEKDAY	RUN (DISTANCE @ RBE)		
1	Sunday	60 min @ 51		
2	Monday	0–30 min @ 51		
3	Tuesday	40–50 min @ 51		
4	Wednesday	10–15 min @ 51		
		1.5 min @ 31 1.5 min @ 51	run 6 to 8 times	
		10–15 min @ 51		
5	Thursday	20–30 min @ 51		
6	Friday	0		
7	Saturday	20 min @ 51		
8	Sunday	10 min @ 51 **RACE:** Marathon 10 min @ 51 or walk		
9	Monday	20–40 min @ 51		
10	Tuesday	0–20 min @ 51		
11	Wednesday	20–30 min @ 51		
12	Thursday	30–40 min @ 51		
13	Friday	10–20 min @ 51		
14	Saturday	0		

Rhythmic Runner:
Jon Keagy

RUNNER PROFILE: took up running in 2007; PRs include 19:36 for 5-K, 1:33:59 for half-marathon, and 3:28:17 for marathon

AGE: 46

OCCUPATION: electrical engineer

> "With rhythmic breathing, I run a more even effort and finish stronger in my races."

Jon Keagy didn't take up running until he was 41 and never considered himself a runner until people referred to him as one. He ran his first race—a 5-K—in March 2008 and was hooked. Since then he's completed more than 30 races from the 5-K to the marathon. One day, Keagy's weekend training group said to him, "There are two types of runner: those who have run Boston and those who want to run Boston." A fire was lit in Keagy's belly.

He put together a training plan and ran the Richmond Marathon in Boston-qualifying time. But then Boston changed its standards for 2012. Keagy had to run another, faster marathon. "I decided to get some professional advice, and a friend introduced me to Budd Coates," he says. The two met for a run, and Coates explained rhyth-

mic breathing and its benefits.

In his enthusiasm for the sport, Keagy subscribes to *Runner's World* magazine and has devoured several books on training, but nowhere had he come across information about how best to breathe during training and racing. He eagerly adapted rhythmic breathing to his workouts.

Focusing on breathing has made Keagy's 20-mile training runs easier, and pacing has become simpler and more controlled. "I have a GPS watch, but now I use my breathing to determine my pace and make sure I am running at the right effort.

"With rhythmic breathing, I run a more even effort and finish stronger in my races," he adds. In April 2012, Keagy joined the ranks of those who have run that hallowed race.

CHAPTER 10

TRAINING ON HILLS

"If the hill has its own name, then it's probably a pretty tough hill."—Marty Stern

I n my 30-plus years living in Emmaus, Pennsylvania, I have discovered hills on grass, road, and trails that allow me to do workouts quite similar to those Arthur Lydiard used in New Zealand more than 50 years ago in his own training and with his athletes. One of my most memorable experiences occurred one weekend in the fall of 1995 when I hosted Arthur during one of his US tours. I drove him over almost every one of my hill courses. One loop in particular offered a variety of courses from 5 miles to 19 and even, much to Arthur's delight, a 22-mile option. The smile on his face was a stamp of approval—not so much for the courses themselves but for the fact that I had taken his principles and applied them to the countryside around my home and was sharing them with others.

Despite Lydiard's being heralded as one of the greatest long-distance coaches of all time, current coaches and exercise physiologists have long debated whether runners need to include hill training in their running programs and, if so, just how it should be incorporated. With regard to specificity of training, most will agree that if your goal race includes hills, your training should as well. But many share the view of a teammate of mine from Springfield College who would say, "No hills on the track—no hills in my training."

My experience and observations over 30 years of racing and coaching have shown that the strength you develop from running uphill and the resilience (through the eccentric contractions of muscles) you gain from running downhill will pay dividends no matter what the distance or hilliness of your goal race.

Hills, Physiology, and Biomechanics

Consider the positive impact hill training has on your body's fitness. Physiologically, hills force you to work harder because when you're training on them you're not just moving your body forward, you're also moving it up against gravity. This increases the workload on your glutes, quads, and calves, and you fatigue sooner than you do when running on a flat course. But as you adapt, you become stronger. And hills deliver a biomechanical benefit as well. You lift your knees higher, you bend farther at the hip, and, with full foot contact on the ground, you increase the motion of your ankle. You're working all of your running muscles in a greater range of motion than ever before. Increased strength plus greater range of motion leads to a more powerful and longer stride.

And then there's what happens when you come down the other side. Running downhill causes what is called an eccentric contraction. This means that your muscles are contracting but getting longer instead of shorter. Think of it this way—but don't try it: If you were to sit at a leg extension machine (the one in which you sit with your knees bent and ankles behind a padded lever) and lift as much as possible with both legs to a straight-leg position, then quickly drop your left leg while continuing to resist (hold the weight up) with the right, your right leg would slowly bend at the knee and drop down to the starting position. The quadriceps muscle in your right leg would be contracting to hold the weight up but getting longer as it failed and let the weight down. Now let's transfer that to running. Think of your leg as a shock absorber. As you run on flat ground, at footstrike your leg bends at the knee and continues to bend until your quadriceps contracts forcefully enough to straighten your leg and allow you to move forward. During that brief time when your leg is bending farther, your quadriceps is performing an eccentric contraction (contracting but getting longer). When you run downhill, this eccentric contraction is lengthened and causes extra stress to the quads. Yes, you will feel this in delayed-onset

Morning Heart Rate Monitor

As far back as the 1960s, when Fred Wilt was coaching US great Buddy Edelen via airmail letters to England, he used morning heart rate to determine if Buddy was on schedule or overdoing it. An increase of 10 percent in your average morning heart rate means that you are not recovering properly from running and all the stresses you may be facing in your life, making it a valuable tool for assessing training increases and keeping them to an appropriate level.

Here's how it works: When you wake up, continue to lie in bed. Find your pulse and, to ensure accuracy, count it for a full minute. Record the result in your training log or daily planner. Do this every day. Your pulse should stay about the same day after day. A couple of beats' difference once in a while is nothing to be concerned about, but if your pulse has increased for a few days in a row, consider easing up a bit on your harder days. A 10 percent increase means you need to back your training down to a few easy days—including a day off. Allow your morning heart rate to return to its normal average before you resume your scheduled training.

muscle soreness, but your body will adapt and get stronger. This adaptation will increase the power of your stride and prepare you for racing on courses that have significant downhill sections, such as the Boston Marathon course.

In your first forays into hill training, running at a rhythmic breathing effort of 51-52 will challenge you enough to improve your strength and range of motion. Once these runs feel routine, faster runs and interval workouts on hills will deliver even greater benefits. And yet there is an even more challenging workout that, when done correctly, can further improve your running. It's called bounding or plyometrics, and it works by exaggerating the mechanics of uphill running.

To perform bounding, find a steady gradual incline 200 to 300 meters long with a few hundred meters of flat surface at the top and bottom. Grass or cinder provides the ideal surface, but I have used pavement during the winter. When bounding, land on your forefoot, allow your heel to come in full contact with the ground, and bend your knee a little farther than usual. Then think recoil: Push off your heel, straighten your leg, and push off your toes in more of an upward than forward motion. (One of the runners I coached once commented that this is a lot of work to go nowhere in a hurry.) Landing toe first, then heel, creates an eccentric contraction in your calves. Allowing your leg to bend a little farther than usual forces your quads and glutes into a deeper eccentric contraction than usual. And then you undo all of that with a forceful liftoff. Sound like fun?

To execute a bounding workout, warm up first, then bound from the bottom of the hill to the top. Do 50 meters of high-knee-lift skipping on the flat surface at the top. Recover with running at a rhythmic breathing effort of 51 for about a minute (roughly 200 meters). Turn around and run a 100-meter surge, then ease back to 51 for the final 100 meters back to the top of the hill. Now run down the hill at 31-32, being careful not to overstride, landing softly on your feet (no pounding or slapping). At the bottom of the hill, recover running at 51 for about 300 meters.

Turn around, do another stride, recover back to the bottom of the hill, and repeat. Start with two repetitions and increase by two each time you do this workout in your training cycle, to a maximum of eight reps. Only seasoned runners who are training at level C or D should attempt bounding.

Whether you bound up hills, run intervals on hills, or simply include a hilly race in your preparation for your goal race, the key to making hills work for your success as a runner is where and how you include them in your training.

Adding Hills to Your Training

If you are a veteran of Schedule A or you've moved up to Schedule B in base training, find courses that include hills and schedule them for days 4, 7, or 10—the days in the cycle that are assigned your more challenging runs. You don't need to run hills on all three days—one or two will do just fine. The hills you run should be runnable, meaning they shouldn't be so steep or long that you end up walking (or close to it). You also should be able to recover from them, as determined by your morning heart rate. (See "Morning Heart Rate Monitor" on page 173.) If an upcoming race includes hills, choose a course that resembles the race course. Find another route that has many small, rolling hills and yet another with perhaps one long but doable hill. Just outside the front door of our Rodale Inc. office in Emmaus, is a 3-kilometer incline up South Tenth Street. Quite a number of our runners use it as their fitness test, or time trial, and it's even been conquered on an ElliptiGO, a cross-training device that combines elements of running, cycling, and the elliptical trainer to deliver a workout that mimics running outdoors while eliminating the impact.

If your choice of hilly routes is limited, consider running the hill courses you do have in the opposite direction. It changes the stresses of the run and the views. Once you enter race-specific training, these hill runs will be replaced with other quality workouts; you may, however, continue to run them on day 7 of your schedule if your goal race includes hills.

If you are a Schedule B veteran or you are using Schedule C or D, you have more options for including hills in your training. You can add them on days 4, 7, or 10, or even tackle a long run over a hilly course as long as the climbs do not interfere with your ability to cover the distance; the purpose of the long run is to spend a long time on your feet, and that purpose is defeated by a shorter workout with hills. Once you shift into race-specific training, you have many choices for using hills as you prepare for your goal race.

- **Option 1:** You can simply replace the hill training with the quality workouts scheduled. The hill running you've done in base training will have taken you to a higher level of fitness than if you had done all or most of your running on flat courses. You'll be able to perform your quality workouts at a higher level and you'll arrive at the starting line of your race better prepared than ever.

- **Option 2:** Step it up a notch and run hills on days allocated for moderate workouts—days 3, 6, and 9 (again, how many hill runs you include is your choice). At first, this may sound daunting—perhaps even foolish—because it means the rhythm of your race training will look like this: long run, easy day, hill run, intervals, easy, hills, tempo, and so forth. But as your fitness improves, what once felt hard now feels easy; those hills that pushed your rhythmic breathing effort up from 51 to 52 and 53 now can be run at 51. Your hill runs have become moderate runs. That being said, don't take these increases in training for granted. Make sure you are ready for them and that you are recovering from them. As your training progresses, you adapt to the changes and your fitness increases, but it is possible to overshoot your ability to adapt.

Fortunately, you can easily monitor your training progression by tracking your morning heart rate. (Again, see "Morning Heart Rate Monitor" on page 173.)

- **Option 3:** You may take your quality workouts—intervals—to the hills. Again, progression is the key to success in training and race readiness. Don't throw all of your options into one race-specific schedule—hills on moderate days and on long runs and with intervals. Take it one step at a time, even one race at a time, as your fitness builds.

Hill Training in Action

If you feel ready to include hills in your training, following are detailed examples of how to do so. Track your morning heart rate to make sure you are progressing wisely.

Schedule B Runners

Adding hills to your schedule is simple and produces significant gains in fitness.

- **Phase 1:** In base training, plan to run hilly courses on day 4 and either day 7 or 10.

- **Phase 2:** When you move into race-specific training, find a hill where you can do the long intervals scheduled for day 10 of your training cycles but keep the other quality workouts on level terrain. If the hill turns out to be a little short—say, 10 to 20 seconds short—that's okay; any shorter, though, and you need to find another hill. If, on the other hand, the hill is long, simply turn around at the completion of your interval and jog down for your recovery. As your fitness improves, you'll run farther and farther up the hill during your interval.

- **Phase 3:** Once you reach cycle 4 in race training, begin using flat-ter terrain that allows you to run these intervals at a pace closer to your race pace.

Schedule C and D Runners

You've reached a high level of training and you've logged many miles. And while consistent training at this level will continue to deliver improvements in performance, you may be looking for more. Hill training brings a new challenge and will take your fitness and performance even further. Because you are very fit, you can do more hill training and you have more options than the less experienced runner will, so it is especially important that you follow a smart and calculated progression as you incorporate hills into your workouts. Here's how.

- **Phase 1:** Begin by running hilly courses on the harder days—days 4 and 10—of your base training. Run them at the same rhythmic breathing effort as given in the schedule. However, because the course is more difficult, you will likely be running a slower pace than you are accustomed to. If, at any point, the steepness of the hill forces you from an RBE of 51 to 52 and into 53, slow down and ease your RBE back into the 51-52 range. Always settle into a 51 on the downhill and flat portions of the course. If you run these hills at the appropriate level of effort, your fitness will improve as you progress from training cycle to training cycle and you will be able to run these hills consistently at a 51 RBE.

- **Phase 2:** With the fitness you've gained from running hills during base training, you should be able to move the hill runs to two of your moderate-workout days—days 3, 6, or 9—once you start race-specific training. You will, however, need to shorten these hill runs to match the distance prescribed on your schedule for these days. You may also include some challenging hills in your long run on day 1.

- **Phase 3:** You've been covering hilly terrain on a couple of your moderate days and you may even be including some challenging hills in your long run. As long as you are following your rhythmic breathing effort to ensure that you are running at the right effort level for the purpose of those workouts, you should be ready for the next step. You have two options.

    - **Option 1:** Simply do the interval workouts on days 4 and 10 of your schedule on rolling terrain—nothing that includes hills longer than about 400 to 600 meters (¼ to ⅜ of a mile) and roughly a 7 percent grade (4 degrees, or 1 meter of climb every 14 meters).

    - **Option 2:** Find hills that you can use to create workouts such as the ones that follow. Some runners refer to these as hill repeats. They will replace the long intervals listed for days 4 and 10.

Following is a Lydiard hill workout that's perfect for day 4 of your schedule. It requires a long, gradual hill of about 1,000 meters (½ mile will do). My favorite surface for these is grass, but I also have road options for winter months. Lydiard's original course for this workout was "around the block," meaning that his athletes would run uphill hard, recover while running across the block to the downhill section, run the downhill hard, and then recover on the return to the start. Runners could choose to do strides within the recovery portions. I've found loops similar to this, but such a course is rare. You will most likely have to run up and down the same hill. Here's what my version of Lydiard hills looks like.

15–20 minutes @ 51 RBE	
150 meters uphill @ 32 150 meters downhill @ 51	2–4 times
1,000 meters uphill @ 31 400 meters @ 51 400–500 meters downhill @ 31 200 meters @ 51	2–4 times
150 meters uphill @ 32 150 meters downhill @ 51	2–4 times
15–20 minutes at 51 RBE	

Following is a bounding workout that you can do on day 10.

15–20 minutes @ 51	
200–300 meters uphill bounding 200 meters flat @ 51 (top of hill) 100 meters flat @ 31 100 meters flat @ 51 200–300 meters downhill @ 31 200 meters flat @ 51 100 meters flat @ 31 100 meters @ 51	2–8 times
15–20 minutes at 51	

And if you are still hungry for hills, you can run a short-hill workout on day 13 of your schedule. I created the following workout to fit one of my favorite running spots. Not far from my home is a small grove of trees planted in rows. It's about ¼ mile square and rests on a hillside. The perimeter and the wide paths between the trees are mowed. It's a great place to run in rhythm with nature.

15 minutes @ 51			
200 meters uphill @ 31-32 80 meters flat @ 51			
80 meters flat @ 31 80 meters flat @ 51	4 times	2–4 times	
300 meters downhill @ 31-32 100 meters @ 51			
15–20 minutes @ 51			

Running intervals on hills is one of the most challenging workouts you'll do. Limit them to the first two or three cycles of your race-specific training and then come back down to flat ground for the remaining speed workouts in your schedule so that you can run at close to race pace. The strength and fitness you've gained on the hills will allow you to draw out the most benefit from these flat intervals as you approach race day.

Rhythmic Runner:
Brian Dalek

RUNNER PROFILE: runs for fitness, camaraderie, and endorphins; enjoys racing to compete not with others but with himself

AGE: 26

OCCUPATION: assistant editor, MensHealth.com

"When I feel like I'm slogging through a run in the heat or on a hill, I focus on my breathing and it brings everything together."

Brian Dalek had left his racing days behind him in high school, where he ran track and cross-country, until he moved to Pennsylvania's Lehigh Valley to work for Rodale Inc., where, as a runner, he was soon introduced to Budd Coates. "Budd would oversee intervals on the jogging trail behind the gym every Wednesday and I'd go to the workouts," Dalek says. Running regularly with a group of competitive athletes, Dalek caught the racing bug. He ran a local half-marathon in 1:31 and then in the fall of 2011 finished the Philadelphia Marathon in 3:25.

It was after one of the Wednesday workouts that Dalek and Coates talked about rhythmic breathing. Dalek decided to give it a try and has found it a terrific tool in many ways. "When I feel like I'm slogging through a run in the heat or on a hill, I focus on my breathing and it brings everything together," he says. "I run taller and my stride opens up."

And though most runners, including Dalek, use rhythmic breathing to hold themselves back from going out too fast, Dalek also relies on rhythmic breathing to tell him when he's running too slow. "A mile and a half into a 5-K, if I'm feeling comfortable I'll check my effort. If it's a comfy 52 [on the RBE scale], I'll bump it up a notch," he says. "I don't think my old self would have been able to do that."

CHAPTER 11

RACING

"Do not bother just to be better than your contemporaries or predecessors. Try to be better than yourself."—William Faulkner

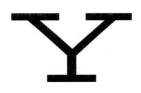our new rhythmic breathing technique not only makes training easier and more effective, it can also improve your race success. One of the most important factors in successful racing is proper pacing. By tuning in to your breathing as soon as the race begins and paying attention to your rhythmic breathing effort, you can run the right pace for the distance. In his paper "The Anticipatory Regulation of Performance," published in the *British Journal of Sports Medicine*, Ross Tucker, PhD, of the University of Cape Town, concludes that, "during exercise, afferent feedback from numerous physiological systems is responsible for the generation of the conscious rate of perceived exertion, which is continuously matched with the subconscious template by means of adjustments in

power output." This means that if you are running a 5-K, your brain will create a template of effort for that distance, which is different from the template it would create for a marathon. You do, however, have some control over your pacing strategy and can adjust it accordingly. In certain race circumstances, you might need to get off the starting line quickly and position yourself up front or out of traffic, but those occasions are rare. For most of us, most of the time, the best strategy is to calmly step into a pace that's appropriate for the race ahead. But the benefits of rhythmic breathing don't end at the start of the race. Used correctly, rhythmic breathing becomes a remarkable strategic tool that can guide you to success at all race distances.

The 5-K

If you're planning to run your first 5-K, your goal should be simply to finish. To guarantee your success in achieving that goal, you need to concentrate on running at an RBE of 51. Remember, as you begin to fatigue toward the end of the race, even though you may be running at the same pace—doing the same amount of work—it won't feel the same; it will feel harder. Your pace at the start may feel like a 51, but that same pace at the end will feel like a 52 or even a 53. Knowing this, you need to make sure your early effort does not feel hard. If you start at a 52 or 53, you'll quickly be forced to convert to a faster 31 RBE, and you may not be experienced or fit enough to maintain that higher level of effort.

Here's the plan: Keep your effort at around 51 during the first mile. Strike up a conversation with your neighboring competitor if you must. As you progress from mile 1 to mile 2, you may notice that your effort is approaching a 52 (you could talk if you wanted to but would rather not). Again, if you're running your first 5-K, I highly recommend that you slow down just a bit so that you can run the last mile at 52 and be assured of a strong finish. But if you get to mile 2 and your breathing effort has simply become too labored, you can move to an RBE of 31 for the final

Hills, Curves, and Competitors

Few race courses offer perfectly even running conditions. You may encounter hills, turns, or U-turns that interrupt your pace. An out-and-back course will likely be windier in one direction. And you may even want to change your pace as a race strategy against your opponents. When your pace and effort are interrupted by course conditions, stay focused on yourself, not the runners around you.

On hills, maintain the rhythmic breathing effort appropriate to that segment of the race, which means you will likely need to slow down a bit. Once you've crested the hill, continue to run at this slower pace for a bit to recover from the climb, then let your pace increase on the downhill while staying in your RBE. Once you reach the bottom of the hill you'll likely need to pull back on the pace a bit to maintain that RBE. Often, runners will hold on to the quicker pace of the downhill and fatigue too early.

Now, if you've done lots of hill training and feel confident that you are really fit, and you want to squeeze out every second possible on the way to the finish line, here's how you do it. At some point on a hill, your rhythmic breathing effort is going to approach 33. Try not to let this happen before the midpoint of the hill (or at least not more than $\frac{1}{2}$ mile from the top of a long hill). Then, rather than slow down so you can run at a 31 or 32, increase your breathing to 2:1:1:1 and hold your effort. Hang in there through the peak of the hill and then relax into the downhill, allowing your effort to return to a 31. You'll recover from the climb to the top and be able to take advantage of gravity on the descent.

For races with lots of turns, gradually decrease your pace going into the turn and gradually increase coming out. The less dramatic your changes in pace, the better. Quick changes create quick and strenuous contractions in your muscles, which can lead to early fatigue.

Surges can be used to advantage in your race strategy against competitors. Frank Shorter, gold medalist in the marathon at the 1972 Olympics, once said that "races are often a series of surges, and the winners of the race are those who can recover from them best." During a race, you or your opponent may put on a strategic surge for a period of time. You need to determine how long you can comfortably handle this change in pace before slowing to your rhythmic breathing effort for this segment of the race. Running too fast or too long will create excessive fatigue and drag down your performance. Practice surges in training. During a tempo run, after you've been running at 52-31 for at least 10 minutes, pick up the effort to a 32-33, hold it for 1 minute, then ease back to 52-31. Put two or three surges into your tempo runs and then use this tactic in your racing.

mile. A 3-count pattern allows you to increase the number of breaths you take per minute.

The experienced 5-K racer can be a bit gutsier. You've been using the faster 3-count breathing pattern in training and in previous races, and you have a good understanding of how long you can perform at a given RBE. So start out at a 31. About a minute into the race, when the runners around you have begun to settle down, change your breathing pattern back to a 5-count pattern for just a few seconds. Don't slow your pace; change your breathing pattern. If, for that short time, the effort feels like a 52—not a 53, where you're breathing as deeply as possible—you are at a good pace and can maintain that pace as you switch back to a 31. If, on the other hand, those few seconds feel like a 53, you need to slow down a bit as you return to the 3-count pattern and an RBE of 31.

If the race course is flat, ideally you will run a consistent pace from start to finish. Use your time at the first mile to confirm that your perceived effort matches your pace, taking into account the environmental conditions. Ask yourself, Can I run at this effort for another 2 miles? And don't hesitate to slow down if the answer is no. It's psychologically harder for most of us to slow down than it is to keep running too fast, but the harder choice is often the right choice.

Check in again at 2 miles. In the perfect race, you feel strong but you

Befriend the Race Course

Arnold Palmer once said, "You must make the golf course your friend." What he meant by that is to play *with* the course, not against it. The same holds true for the runner and the race course. Work from your strengths on the course. If you're a good uphill runner but struggle on the downhill, run the uphills a little faster and relax coming down. Others may find the opposite works best for them. Learn what you're good at in training, and if you can, train on a course similar to that of your upcoming race. Then go enjoy your perfect performance.

are running at an RBE of 32-33. You are working your butt off, but you feel confident that you can hold that effort for the final 1.1 miles. If you are sucking air in like there's no tomorrow, slow down a bit and alter your breathing to a 2:1:1:1 (inhale for two steps, exhale for one, inhale one, exhale one, and repeat). This change increases breaths per minute and, combined with a slower pace, should get you to the finish. If, at the 2-mile mark, your RBE still feels like the 31-32 you ran in the first mile, you can up the ante just a bit. Over the next 1 to 2 minutes, gradually increase your pace by pushing your rhythmic breathing effort toward 33. Don't suddenly drop the pace—you want to ease into this top-end speed and not overstep it.

Now it's time to finish this race, and here's a strategic tip (if you don't already know it): Before the start of the race, jog from the finish line toward the 2-mile mark for 2 minutes and make a mental note of where that is; find a landmark—a house or a store. This is the spot where you will begin to make your finishing surge. At this point, you convert to a 2:1:1:1 breathing pattern and, over the next 30 seconds to 1 minute, increase your pace to a *near* all-out run. Remember, as you fatigue, your pace will feel harder; so if you approach an all-out effort with 100 to 200 yards to go, it'll feel like an all-out effort at the finish line.

The 10-K

Most likely you will have run a few 5-Ks before you decide to move up to the 10-K, and if you've run 5-Ks using the rhythmic breathing strategy discussed above, you will be well prepared for this race distance. I like to divide the 10-K into five segments. The first is from the start to mile 2. You'll race this segment very much as you would the first mile of the 5-K, except that you need to be a bit more cautious. Start at a 31 RBE and, as with the 5-K, at about a minute into the race, change your breathing to the 5-count pattern to make sure you're running under control. Be honest in your assessment: If you aren't sure whether you're at 52 or 53, slow down a bit. Switch back to a 3-count breathing pattern and a 31 RBE. Repeat this pace check at miles 1, 1½, and 2.

At mile 2, your choices are the same as at the 1-mile mark of the 5-K. Can you run 4 more miles at this effort? If the answer is yes, maintain your pace, checking it every ½ mile to the 4-mile mark. If the answer is

Adapting to the Environment

There's nothing more disappointing than having trained to run your best race ever and then having race day arrive with blistering heat and humidity or some other seemingly malicious act of Mother Nature. Here's how to battle through it.

For the 5-K, start out running at an RBE of 52 and allow yourself to increase to a 53. Yes, that's right—53, where you begin to gasp for breath as you run. If done gradually over the first ½ mile, you will be adapting your effort with the environment in check. Then convert your breathing to a 3-count pattern and a 31 RBE, but don't change your pace. You are now inhaling 60 breaths per minute, versus the 36 per minute you inhaled running at 53. As you become fatigued, this same pace will feel like a 32 RBE. If this happens before the 2-mile mark, slow down to bring the effort down to 31. In extreme weather conditions, stay at this pace and effort through to the finish or take it down even further. If climate conditions are moderate and you feel good, you can pick up your effort to a 32 at 2 miles and a 33 when the finish is in sight, but not before 2½ miles. Immediately after the race, jog slowly or walk for 5 to 10 minutes.

At longer race distances, paying attention to your rhythmic breathing effort will be far more valuable to your race success than checking your pace and time on the digital clocks along the course. And this is especially true when the environment makes your pace and the physical work of running feel harder than it should. Heat and humidity increase the demand on the body's cooling systems, so bloodflow gets diverted to the skin, leaving less for your running muscles. You need to adjust your pace, effort, and expectations to meet those constraints. And it's better to err on the low end of your rhythmic breathing effort early on (with the hope that you might be able to increase your pace and effort later) than to be overzealous off the start and fade on the way to the finish line. Or, worse yet, not finish at all.

no, slow down and run at a more relaxed 31, continuing to check your pace every ½ mile.

At 4 miles, you're two-thirds of the way home. Check your pace as before, switching to the 5-count breathing pattern. If your RBE is a solid 52, ask yourself if you can run a little bit faster for 2 more miles or if you should stay where you are. It's a tough question to answer; the more race experience you have, the easier it becomes. If you decide to pick up the pace, make a slight change and make it gradually—aim for an RBE of 32. If you feel fatigue is starting to set in and you're already at a 32 RBE, back off a bit and reassess at 5 miles.

At the 5-mile mark, you have the same choices that the 5-K runner has at 2 miles. If you are running at an RBE of 32-33, are feeling strong, and are confident that you can hold that effort for the final 1.2 miles, maintain your pace and breathing. If you are struggling to breathe, slow down and alter your breathing pattern to a 2:1:1:1 (inhale for two steps, exhale for one, inhale for one, exhale for one, and repeat). Finally, if at the pace you are running the effort is in the 31-32 RBE range, increase your effort over the next 1 to 2 minutes toward 33.

Finish as you would the 5-K. If you have run a consistent pace or were able to increase your pace, you are ready to kick it in from the 6-mile mark, if there is one, or from the point you've identified on the course for the start of your surge. (See The 5-K, page 183.) Switch to a 2:1:1:1 rhythmic breathing pattern and, over the next minute, pick up the pace to a *near* all-out effort and head for the finish line.

15-K through the Half-Marathon

Some runners and coaches treat the 15-K more like a 10-K than a half-marathon, and that's fine for the seasoned runner who has been training and racing for a long time. I believe less-experienced runners should approach the 15-K as they would a half-marathon.

If this is your first venture into longer distances, your goal should be to finish strong. Start the race at an RBE of 51 just as you do your long runs, and maintain that effort for at least two-thirds of the distance. If you feel fresh at that point, increase your pace by raising your effort to a 52 and then move up to a 31 for the final miles of the race. The shift from

The Limits to Performance

If you have raced often, then you likely have experienced some impediment to your best effort—whether that be heat and humidity, fatigue, under-training, overtraining. A multitude of factors—both internal and external—affect physical performance. Exercise physiologist Timothy Noakes gathers them all in the following excerpt from a paper published in April 2012 in the journal series *Frontiers*. That lucky race singlet? You just might want to hold on to it.

> According to this model, exercise begins with feed-forward motor output to recruit the appropriate number of motor units in the exercising muscles. The extent of this recruitment will be determined by a host of factors including, but not exclusively, the biological state of the athlete at the start of exercise, including the emotional state, the extent of mental fatigue, or sleep deprivation, the state of recovery from a previous exercise bout, the level of motivation and prior experience, the degree of self-belief including superstitious beliefs. Factors specific to the event that alter performance include monetary reward, prior knowledge of the exercise end-point, and the presence of competitors, especially if they are of similar ability. A number of chemical agents including the stimulants—amphetamine, caffeine, pseudoephedrine, modafinil, and the dopamine/noradrenaline reuptake inhibitor bupropion—as well as the analgesic acetaminophen, or the analgesic naloxone, or the cytokines interleukin-6, or brain IL-1β have all been shown to alter exercise performance as do placebos. Psychological skills training or pre-exercise whole body cooling can also improve subsequent exercise performance.

> Exercise then begins at an intensity that the brain has determined can be sustained for the expected duration of the exercise bout. As a result all forms of exercise are submaximal since there is always a reserve of motor units in the exercising limbs that is never fully utilized even during maximal exercise especially when undertaken at altitude.

—From "Fatigue is a brain-derived emotion that regulates the exercise behavior to ensure the protection of whole body homeostasis," by Timothy David Noakes, published in *Frontiers in Striated Muscle Physiology*, April 11, 2012.

52 to 31 is only to allow yourself more breaths per minute—keep the pace the same.

Those who have raced longer distances and whose goal is to run a 15-K or 10-miler or half-marathon as fast as their fitness allows can be more aggressive. At the start, go out at a 31 RBE for the first 1 or 2 minutes just to get off the line, but then relax your pace by switching to the 5-count breathing pattern and a 52 RBE. Hold this effort for about 2 more minutes and then, without changing your pace, convert to a 3-count breathing pattern and a 31 breathing effort. The 2 minutes at 52 will cause you to run a little slower at 31 than you would in a 5-K or 10-K and will keep your running under control for the longer distance. At each mile, check your pace by returning to the 5-count breathing pattern for 20 to 30 seconds. If the effort feels like a 53, you are going too fast and need to slow down.

When you've completed two-thirds of the race, check your effort and pace. If you're feeling strong, pick up the pace slightly. But if in doubt—don't. You need to feel sure that you can maintain a greater effort for the remaining miles before you move up to that effort. Wait another mile and again consider whether or not to pick up the pace, and so on to the finish.

As with the shorter races, you will want to locate your point of final attack before the race start by jogging from the finish back along the course for 2 minutes. Once you reach that point in the race, shift up to a 2:1:1:1 RBE if you are able, and put forth a *near* all-out effort, which will feel like an all-out effort as you cross the finish line.

The Marathon

This is the farthest distance you likely will ever run in your life, and if it's your first, your goal should be to finish and be able to talk about it. Start at a pace that corresponds to a 51 RBE and maintain that pace to the finish. Remember, as you fatigue, the effort will feel harder—like a 52 RBE—even though your pace is the same. Ideally, that change in effort from 51 to 52 won't occur until mile 20, preferably mile 22. If it happens sooner, you should slow down immediately. After years of running and coaching, I've come to hold the following to be true: When running the marathon, if you go out too fast, you have no control over how slow you will finish. But if you go out slow, you have total control over how fast you finish. This applies both to those new to this distance as well as the best marathoners in the world.

The experienced marathoner hoping to run a personal best or to qualify for Boston should also start at an RBE of 51 and within the first few minutes ease into a 52. Your first success will be in not paying any attention to those other runners who are passing you. Once you are comfortably cruising along at 52, keep your pace the same but convert to a 31 RBE. The plan is to continue at this effort and pace until you reach the 15-mile point, but check your pace and effort at each mile. Switch back to a 5-count breathing pattern at your current pace, and if the effort is comfortably a 52, revert to 31 and run steady on. If the effort is a 53, meaning you can't talk, slow down immediately. Wesley Korir, winner of the 2012 Boston Marathon and runner-up at the Chicago Marathon in 2011, said of the early miles in his 2:06:15 performance at Chicago, "During the race we were praying and singing and talking, and it was just so much fun."

In a story addressing the US marathon qualifiers for the 2012 Olympic Games (*Runner's World* magazine, August 2012), former Olympian Don Kardong advised the runners to dissociate during the first half of the race, to run on autopilot and let the mind wander. Then it becomes time to associate; focus on your goal; monitor your breathing, fatigue, and other variables—aches and pains, weather, terrain, competition—and make whatever adjustments are necessary to achieve that goal.

I'm not sure who was first to coin this phrase, but the marathon has often been described as a "20-mile jog followed by a 10-K race." It's an apt description, because the fact is, run correctly, the marathon *feels* like that even though the pace often doesn't change—or at least changes very little. Don't forget (as if I would let you) that as fatigue from the first 20 miles sets in, perceived exertion increases, making the same pace feel more like a race

Racing the Boilermaker

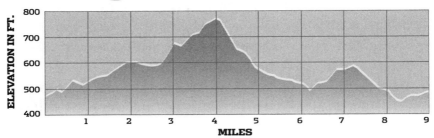

Budd's elevation graph for the Boilermaker.

The Utica Boilermaker is a 15-K road race held every July just a few miles from my hometown of Camden in central New York State. Running this race has become a family tradition, and in 2012 (while writing this book) I shared the experience with my wife, my daughter, three nephews, a niece, and a cousin.

The elevation graph tells it all—this 15-K travels challenging terrain, and the race is made even more difficult by July's heat. I started at a rhythmic breathing effort of 31, regularly checking my pace. This led me through 3 miles with split times close to 6:30 for each mile.

At about 3.5 miles, well into the climb, I could feel the effort approach 33. Because I knew I was close to the top of the hill, I opted to shift to 2:1:1:1 (faster breathing/more breaths per minute) rather than slow down to a 31, because I knew that once I was over the top, I could recover at 31 and cruise down the hill.

I had gone through the 5-K point slower than I had hoped to (20:08), but at 4 miles I felt confident that I could now take advantage of the rest of the course. I stayed as relaxed as possible on the descent but still slipped through that 4th mile in close to 5 minutes. Maintaining a 31, I slowed a bit but ran well through 6 miles. Checking the clock, I had run the second 5-K in 18:30.

Now to climb the next hill. Just as before, my effort intensified to 33, and again I opted to shift to the 2111 breathing pattern to crest the hill without slowing. It was difficult, and it took longer to recover, but once I did, I was on my way to the finish.

I had been steadily passing other runners for the first 7 miles, but now—not so often. I keyed on three runners a hundred or so yards in front of me and kept running at a hard 33-2:1:1:1 RBE. At mile 9, it was time to let it all out and run at 2:1:1:1. I caught the three runners with 50 yards to go, which gave one of them enough time to then catch me back. But I finished in just over 57 minutes, had run the final 5-K in another 18:30, and won the over-55 title.

than it did during the early miles. In addition, these changes in rhythmic breathing effort (or perceived exertion) occur at a faster and higher level than in shorter races, because you've been on your feet for a long time, accumulating fatigue and burning up your source of energy (glucose).

So what does that mean? It means that your 51-52 rhythmic breathing effort will progress all the way to a 33 even though you are not running any faster. Your job as an experienced runner is to prevent that from happening until at least 22 or 23 miles. Assess your effort and pace at each mile as I've described earlier. If you think you can continue at that pace to the finish, carry on with it. If you don't think you can maintain that pace, slow down just a bit and return to a 3-count breathing pattern and 31 RBE. This new pace should carry you through to the finish. If you ignore your fatigue and continue to push on at the faster pace, you will most likely "hit the wall" and slow down more than you ever thought possible. The "wall" is an unfortunate combination of miles of pounding plus having run a pace that exhausts you, metabolizing all of your glycogen and glucose.

Once you've reached mile 22 or 23, it's time to start repeating the mantra "Here I come" until you see the finish line, at which point you can start saying "Here I am."

Finally

Very few of us will ever run the perfect race—but we can come close. Every runner is different. Every race is different. Every race day is different. You will take something from every race you run. You will learn your limits, your strengths, and your ability to perform at given rhythmic breathing efforts. Apply this knowledge to your next phase of training and to your next race, and you'll reap the rewards. As you gain more experience racing with rhythmic breathing, it becomes second nature. You will need to focus less on those early-mile breathing and pace checks and instead allow yourself to dissociate and simply run.

Rhythmic Runner:
Kathleen Jobes

PROFILE: competitive masters runner; top female in masters division at 2012 Chicago Marathon with a time of 2:47; competed in the US Olympic Marathon Trials in 2008; coached by Steve Jones

AGE: 42

OCCUPATION: integrated marketing director

> "Rhythmic breathing brought me consistency in pacing and helped me PR. It is the best thing I've ever learned."

A fierce and hungry competitor, Kathleen Jobes would simply devour the road in front of her as she leapt off the starting line, but running too fast too soon would force her to a disappointing finish. At the next event she'd rein in her fervor, but a conservative effort also would cost her a top performance. "I was terrible at pacing myself during races," Jobes says. "I'd go out too fast or too slow. I had no idea what effort I was running at."

Budd Coates suggested she try rhythmic breathing, then taught her how to do it and how to use it. "I started using rhythmic breathing in 2006," says Jobes. "Now I know what effort I'm at and whether or not I'm running the right pace. If I'm in a 1:1 pattern, I know I need to drop back to 2:1." Jobes went on to compete in the 2008 US Olympic Marathon Trials, and at 42 she won the women's masters division at the 2012 Chicago Marathon in a time of 2:47.

"I used to have so much anxiety that I'd go out too fast," says Jobes. "Now I have control over my running and I am much more relaxed at the start of a race. From a pacing standpoint, rhythmic breathing made me consistent and helped me PR. It is the best thing I've ever learned." And as a competitive masters runner, Jobes continues to improve and is very close to going back under 17 minutes in the 5-K.

CHAPTER 12

CROSS-TRAINING

"Every day, in every way, I am getting better and better."—Emile Coue

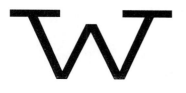hen I was at Springfield College in the '70s, most schools didn't have facilities where athletes could do supplementary training—cross-training, in today's terminology. So when I was injured—which, if you recall, was often—I would head to the exercise physiology building, where Dr. A.J. "Jack" Mahurin gave me permission to use one of the Monarch test bikes. I asked Jack what sort of workout I should do and he said, "Do whatever the team is doing today." With that very good advice I pedaled away, without music or TV, just an old poster of how the Krebs cycle worked in front of me.

Of course, the best way to become a better runner is to run—it trains your muscles and cardiovascular and respiratory systems in the exact work you need them to do when you run. But there are occasions when cross-training can be very valuable to a runner. When you're injured, cross-training maintains your conditioning. (Did I mention that it's easier to stay fit than to get fit?) And if you are susceptible to injury, including cross-training in your running regimen may help you avoid getting hurt. Some runners like the variety of mixing in cycling, swimming, or another activity among their running workouts. For me, well, as I've gotten older and "softer," I sometimes opt for indoor cross-training options on days when it's particularly cold, windy, rainy, or all of the above.

Rhythmic Breathing in Cross-Training

The runner who uses the rhythmic breathing method of training has an advantage over other runners when turning to cross-training to maintain conditioning. Remember Jack's advice? "Do whatever the team is doing today." By applying rhythmic breathing efforts (RBEs) to whatever cross-training activity you choose, you can replicate the effort you would be exerting on the run that you had planned for that day. Let's say you are scheduled to do a workout of six to eight 2-minute fast repeats. Here's how that would look on an elliptical trainer or stairclimber:

1. Exercise at an RBE of 51 for 10 minutes (the warmup).

2. Increase the effort to 31 (by changing the pace and/or resistance) for 2 minutes.

3. Bring the effort back down to 51 (change the pace or resistance) for 1 minute.

4. Repeat 2 minutes hard/1 minute easy for a total of 6 to 8 repetitions.

5. Do a 10-minute cooldown by bringing your exercise level down to a 51.

You can do a similar workout on a stationary bike or while cycling outdoors. Ride comfortably for the warmup; cycle in a standing position for 2 minutes at a 31 RBE; sit and spin at 51 for 1 minute and repeat for a total of 6 to 8 reps; then cool down for 10 minutes at a 51 RBE.

Cross-Training Options

You have more cross-training options available to you than ever before, including swimming, cycling (indoor or out), elliptical machines, stair-climbers, and rowers. Swimming will demand that you breathe rhythmically, although inhalation and exhalation occur in sync with your stroke cadence, not your stride, as they do in running. Rowing requires a different breathing pattern altogether. But with other activities, you can easily apply rhythmic breathing.

Elliptical Training

When elliptical trainers arrived in the 1990s, they became the runner's choice for cross-training because, of all activities, elliptical training most closely resembles the motions of running, and the stride cadence is quite similar. This similarity in stride cadence means that the rhythmic breathing patterns are a natural fit. You can mount yourself on an elliptical and do the exact same workout you had planned for an outdoor run.

Life got even better when the ElliptiGO was born. I refer to it—all in fun—as the grasshopper, for obvious reasons. The ElliptiGO offers the injured runner an opportunity to log some very specific outdoor training. And it allows the often-injured runner to enjoy the outdoors while getting a break from pounding the roads. It's safest to use ElliptiGOs on the road or on paved trails, though some very able-bodied individuals are adept at using them on more challenging surfaces, such as grass.

Stairclimbing

Though stairclimbing and running have biomechanical differences, the similarities make stairclimbing a good cross-training choice for runners. Most stairclimbers work against your body weight. As the readout on the screen indicates, at a higher and higher work level, the pedals resist your weight less and less, and you must step faster and faster so as not to bottom out and hit the floor. This means that at a low level of work, your cadence is slow; and at a high level of work, your cadence is faster. Since the typical running cadence is between 180 and 200 strides per minute regardless of how fast you are running, you need to figure out what level on the stairclimber allows you to do at least 180 steps a minute to most closely replicate running. A slower stair workout is sufficient for an easy or moderate day, but for an interval or tempo workout, you want to be as close to your running cadence as possible to use your rhythmic breathing efforts effectively.

Cycling

Stationary bikes have come a long way from the old Monarch test bikes that I used during my early injury-prone days as a runner, but cycling still has limitations as a cross-training activity for runners. As we've already mentioned, the natural cadence for a runner is about 180 to 200 steps per minute. While cycling, you'll spin at a much faster rate— spinning at 180 to 200 cycles per minute while sitting on a bike is simply too slow to create any meaningful effort. As a runner, you have few options for working out at the appropriate effort.

If you are planning a long, easy, or moderate run, simply spin at a rate that requires an easy pace at which you can talk comfortably. You may, however, want to get out of the saddle for 30 to 60 seconds every 10 minutes or so just to get off your butt.

If quality is the purpose of the day's run, then during the speed portion of the workout you need to increase the resistance on the bike, get up out of the saddle, and "run on your bike." That's right, run on your bike. You can do this in a couple of different ways.

1. On a stationary bike, increase the resistance, stand, and spin at about 180 to 200 cycles per minute while using the 3-count breathing pattern and a 31 RBE for the specific time interval required of that day's workout. Sit, release the resistance, and spin for the length of the recovery. I refer to this as "sit 'n' spin" in the indoor classes that I've taught. Repeat as necessary. Research tells us that the best indoor workout is intervals of 3 minutes in the standing position followed by 3 minutes seated.

2. Outside, you can do the same workout just described for stationary bikes, or you can find a hilly loop. Stand and spin at least 180 cycles per minute on the uphills; sit and spin on the downhills and flat sections. You can go back and forth on the same hill for an interval workout or find a longer loop with a variety of inclines.

Though you will never be able to get the exact workout on the bike that you had scheduled for your run, you can come close, and one of the goals of cross-training is to maintain overall fitness. On your easy and moderate days, simply spin for the time you would have been running. Quality workouts can mimic the effort you would have run in training, but remember, a 3-minute interval on a bike will take you a lot farther (distance) than while running, and you'll be going a lot faster. Be careful not to overdo it.

Mini-Trampoline

I have owned a mini-trampoline for over 30 years and have run on it countless times while nursing an injury, as have almost all of my running friends. It doesn't make any noise. It's easy to stow away. It's easy to toss into the car and deliver to a friend or take on vacation. And it serves the purpose quite well. Though the give in the trampoline makes it difficult to get up to that minimum of 180 strides per minute, you can come close and you can apply your rhythmic breathing efforts to each workout. To achieve a rhythmic breathing effort of 51, lift your feet and knees very little. Lifting your feet and knees higher increases the work and consequently your RBE. You can train on the mini-tramp with almost any injury (but not every one). It's a great comeback tool.

Swimming

I challenge anyone reading this book to a worst-swimmer contest and I bet I'll win. I know my wife, daughter, son, and all my friends would put their money on me. Even John McVan, my swim coach from years ago, would bet on me. That being said, swimming is a great cross-training option for runners. Swimming forces you to use rhythmic breathing, though you do so via your stroke cadence.

You can complete a long or easy workout simply by swimming lap after lap for the length of your prescribed run. If a quality workout is on tap, swim harder for a lap or two and then rest at the pool's edge, or swim an easier stroke for the recovery period between hard laps.

Mastering breathing during swimming can be a challenge for runners, and for some individuals it causes extreme neck discomfort. Swimming with a snorkel solves these issues and allows you to swim comfortably from one end of the pool to the other.

By using a snorkle, you can apply rhythmic breathing to your swim workouts but with a slight twist. Stroke rate for most people is too slow to use a 5-count breathing pattern (inhale for three strokes, exhale for two), so you will probably need to use the 3-count pattern (inhale for two strokes, exhale for one). For long, easy, and moderate workouts, swim at a 31 RBE. For tempo runs and long intervals, warm up at 31 and move up to 32 for the quality work. The 2:1:1:1 rhythmic breathing pattern will work for short, fast intervals. You will most definitely go through a trial-and-error period as you learn to master rhythmic breathing during swimming, but hang in there, you'll love the results.

Pool Running

Running in the pool is certainly mechanically more aligned to running than swimming, but I—much to your surprise, I'm sure—would rather swim. That said, I've run in the pool with buoyant vests and belts but recommend that you go without either. Use your arm carriage and running stride to keep you afloat. You'll work a bit harder, but it's doable. Because you are using a running stride, you can replicate your scheduled land workout in the water.

Rowing

If you have a rowing background, you were most likely taught one of a number of breathing techniques. For the purposes of cross-training, let's keep it simple. Rowing has two motions—the pull and the return. Exhale during the pull and inhale on the return. To relate your rowing effort to your running effort, use this scale: 1—easy rowing (RBE 51-52); 2—moderate rowing (RBE 52-31); and 3—hard rowing (RBE 32-33).

On the Road Again

When your injury has healed and you are ready to return to running, start back with base training and complete the Schedule A, 14-day cycle regardless of what schedule you were using when you suffered your injury. If you were training at Schedule A, however, cut each run by 50 percent. If you have a race coming up and need to prepare, use cross-training for your quality workouts.

Once you can say that you are 100 percent pain-free and very comfortable with the running in the Schedule A base-training cycle, you can move up in training. The Schedule A runner can progress to the full

Schedule A base training or the Schedule A race-specific training. *All* other runners move to Schedule B with quality workouts. Schedule B runners may choose to use cross-training for the quality workouts on the first run through this cycle. If you're a Schedule C runner, you should complete this cycle once and then move up to Schedule C training, running the lower end of the range for distance and intervals and increasing within those ranges only if you can say absolutely and with 100 percent honesty that you are healthy enough for more. If you were running on Schedule D prior to your injury, complete the Schedule C cycle twice before returning to D-level training.

Cross-training alone will not keep you in race shape, but it can help maintain overall conditioning and fitness so that when you return to running you are physically strong and ready to go. My go-to podiatrist, Dr. Neal Kramer, always cautioned me about getting back on the road after an injury. He'd say, "Budd, I know you've been keeping yourself incredibly fit during this time off, but make sure you ease back into actual running."

Cross-training limits the big loss in fitness that would come with sitting on the couch watching *Mad Men* reruns. And perhaps that hiatus from running will spark your enthusiasm for feeling your feet on the roads and trails again and make you hungry for the sport. But it's a bit like the marathon: If you go out too fast, you'll pay the price.

Rhythmic Runner:
Kristie Fach

RUNNER PROFILE: ran competitively in high school and college; increased mileage postcollege to train for the half-marathon and marathon

AGE: 35

OCCUPATION: biologist for a land trust

"For years I would have pain in every step and turn when running around with my boys. With rhythmic breathing, I was able to go for a bike ride with them—pain-free."

Most runners use rhythmic breathing to prevent injury. Kristie Fach is using it to recover from one. In 2006, Fach experienced a cramp on her right side underneath her lower ribs—an injury that marked the onset of a sharp pain in the abdominal area under her ribs that would flare with every breath. She continued running an average of 70 miles a week for several months, until the pain was too much to bear.

After consulting with a variety of doctors and specialists, she learned that a confluence of factors had led to her chronic injury, including mild scoliosis and a tight psoas muscle (which runs from the lower spine through the pelvis to the top of the thighbone). Fach had followed a complex regimen of stretches, exercise, and therapies to resolve her injury but was still unable to run pain-free for any length of time. In the spring of 2012, she met with Budd Coates to discuss if rhythmic breathing might help.

"Budd explained that the greatest impact stress of running occurs at the beginning of exhalation. Since my injury was on my right side, he advised that I exhale as my left foot hit the ground and use a 2:2 pattern of breathing, which would keep the impact on the left and relieve pressure from my injured right side," explains Fach. "I gave it a shot with the ElliptiGO, and I could tell immediately that it took the pressure off.

"Rhythmic breathing helps relax my psoas and allows me to push my breathing more," Fach adds, "and since I've started using it, I haven't had any flare-up of my injury during or after a workout on the ElliptiGO."

Her boys have benefited, too.

"For years I would have pain playing and running around with my boys," says Fach. "With rhythmic breathing, I was able to go for a bike ride with them, pain-free."

Fach is not fully recovered from her injury, but she's much closer. "I have things in place now," she says. "The main work is to loosen up and get stronger." And Fach's grit and determination, combined with the restorative power of breathing, will indeed get her back on the road running and training again—pain-free.

CHAPTER 13

TRAIL RUNNING

**"Two roads diverged in a wood, and I—
I took the one less traveled by,
And that has made all the difference."**

—Robert Frost, "The Road Not Taken"

D uring the spring of my sophomore year in high school, I became friends with a senior on our track team by the name of Mike Wolcott. Mike was a very good runner, but what I remember most was his love of trail running. There were no official walking and running paths near our small town, but there were plenty of marked snowmobile trails that were great to explore on foot from spring through fall. Whenever we could break free from team practice, I would simply follow Mike through the woods, never quite knowing where we were going, just running. In the 40 years since, I haven't lost that love of heading into a local forest.

Not only is trail running enormous fun, it is a much-overlooked training gem that can contribute significantly to your success. A trail run can mean a run on open grass, golf courses, groomed cinder paths, rails-to-trails routes, runnable singletrack footpaths through the woods or up a mountain, rutted, obstacle-filled dirt passages, and, of course, snowmobile trails. This multitude of terrains allows for a variety of training and benefits that can't be accrued on the road or track.

Just about any workout can be performed on a groomed trail or grass, and you'll enjoy the benefits of a softer surface, better scenery, and the absence of traffic lights. But it's the more challenging trails that I find the most valuable and that offer the greatest reward. Rough, uneven trails that wander through the woods and up and down hills force you to keep your pace under control. They may require you to step side to side, climb, descend, jump, walk, or pick your feet up higher. They put you through motions and movements outside of your usual running gait. These movements train a number of auxiliary muscles that when strengthened can help prevent injury. Many coaches prescribe drills that activate auxiliary muscles, but in a recent conversation with Golden Harper, the inventor of Altra running shoes and an avid trail runner, we both agreed we'd rather play

Trail Etiquette

As you begin running off-road, you'll find yourself sharing the trails not only with other runners and walkers but with mountain bikers and horseback riders. Follow these two right-of-way rules:

1. Bikers and runners should stop for those on horseback.

2. Bikers should yield to runners.

As a courtesy to cyclists, however, and to ensure your own safety in the path, I recommend that you step aside and let the cyclist pass.

in the woods than spend 30 minutes inside or out doing a series of drills.

The fear of succumbing to injury discourages many runners from trail running. The fact is, more people turn ankles when an unexpected obstacle or depression appears underfoot during a run on smooth terrain than when venturing onto rugged paths. When you run on rough surfaces, your mind and body become more aware of the unevenness beneath your feet and you naturally fall into a gait and footstrike that will help you avoid injury. While you can never be 100 percent certain that you won't experience some mishap on the trails, the benefits to your running far outweigh the risks.

If you are new to trail running or feel a little cautious about the endeavor, start with a trail that's more varied than a groomed path but that you know won't get too rutted, rocky, and strewn with tree roots. Skip the stream crossings. Go have fun and get fitter along the way.

How to Train on Trails

The most important thing to keep in mind as you move a workout—particularly an easy or moderate one—from a paved or groomed surface to difficult terrain is to run for the same amount of time and at the same effort that you would have run on the road or track. Remember, it's the effort, not the mileage, that matters. If your typical easy 40-minute run takes you over a 5-mile route and you attempt to complete 5 miles of rocky, hilly trails, the run may take far too long and leave you tired for your next workout. Remember to apply the appropriate rhythmic breathing effort. If you are scheduled to run easy, keep your effort at a 51 RBE. For a moderate workout, run no harder than 52. When I hit the trails on an easy day and I encounter a stiff climb that forces me to run beyond a 51, I will walk at 31 until the terrain allows me to run comfortably again. (Yes, it's okay to walk during some workouts.) For quality runs on grass or groomed trail, stay at the appropriate RBE as prescribed on your schedule.

Choosing the Right Trail

Remember, you have many options for trail running, from groomed cinder paths to the rough and rocky. And you have a variety of workouts in your schedule. You always want to get the most training benefit from every workout, even when you go off-road, and that entails picking the best surface for the type of running you will be doing. Here's a look at your different workouts and the best trails for running them.

Quality: long run, long and short intervals, tempo run

To get the most from your quality workouts on the trail, you will need to run them at about the same pace and effort as you would on the road or track. This is not the time to choose a technically difficult trail. You want a surface with smooth, even footing: A cinder path, groomed trail, or grass path will work well. For long runs, choose a route that's similar in its hills and flats to your goal race, especially if you are training for any distance from 15-K to the marathon.

Easy

Easy runs should be just that—easy. This is your recovery day, so head down a path that will allow you to stay consistently in that relaxed 51 RBE. When you go off-road, choose a trail that doesn't vary too much in terrain and that offers smooth and even footing, similar to the type of trail you would use for quality runs. Because the goal is opposite that of

Specificity of Surfaces

A note about training and racing surfaces: If you plan to do some road racing, you must train on roads so that your body adapts to the surface. But that does not mean all of your training needs to be done on the asphalt. Mixing trail running into your schedule will make you a stronger runner and help you avoid injury—and it's fun.

Trail Smarts

Some of the best trail-running experiences are had on paths that carry you deep into the woods, away from civilization, where you can immerse yourself in nature. And as much as you might yearn for a solitary sojourn, you would be wise to travel such trails with a friend or two. You'll likely need to run single file most of the way, so leave about 5 yards between you and the next runner, which will give you a clear view of the trail in front of you. If you must venture out alone, choose a trail that you know is frequented by other runners, mountain bikers, and hikers (just in case you need a friend), and leave word at home as to where you're running and how long you'll be gone.

a quality workout—your purpose is to recover, not to challenge your body—the running surface should support that purpose by allowing the fullest recovery.

Moderate

It's time to play in the woods. Though you still need to run within the correct rhythmic breathing effort for this workout, you have more play in how you do it. You don't need to keep your effort consistently easy, and you don't have to worry about footing that might interrupt your pace and effort for, say, a long interval. Any trail works for the moderate run— even those that cross a stream. (Did I say I had fun in the woods?) And here's where you will reap the greatest rewards of trail running. Challenging trails force you to make just about every move you can imagine. They demand a variety of foot plants and they alter your pace countless times. The only caution: Avoid too steep a hill or climbing for too long. Limit the climb to 2 minutes—and that includes any walking you are forced to do. Remember, the goal is to run these moderate trail runs at a 51 to 52 RBE. A steep climb will likely push you above that and into a walk at 31. A moderate run on trails should leave you feeling refreshingly tired but in good shape for the more serious workout the next day. If it doesn't, choose a different path the next time.

I like to finish these runs with six to ten 100-meter strides in my bare feet on groomed grass—a football or soccer field works well. In fact, I like to do all of my strides barefoot whenever I can find a good surface. My Springfield College teammates and I started doing this in the late '70s. It felt good to let our feet grip the grass beneath them, and we loved how light we felt running without shoes.

Making Tracks

Though paths and trails aren't always convenient, they are worth traveling to with a few friends. Here in the Lehigh Valley we are blessed with a beautiful cinder path along the Little Lehigh Creek that is also home to our local running club, the Lehigh Valley Road Runners. Nearby is the Delaware and Lehigh National Heritage Corridor. There are trails within local land preserves, and not too far away is the Appalachian Trail. When I travel to New York City, I can find soft paths in Central Park and Prospect Park. To find trails near you, check out AllTrails.com. And consider becoming active in creating local trails. In the past few years I have assisted our community in upgrading and creating both singletrack and grass paths. Join efforts with your local mountain bike community. These men and women put in a lot of time grooming trails. And as you begin weaving your runs through the woods, you'll understand why.

Rhythmic Runner:
Kim Draves

RUNNER PROFILE: runs for health and fitness

AGE: 38

OCCUPATION: consumer marketing director for magazines

> "I can control my breathing. I now have a tool that allows me to recover if I go out too fast or if something goofy happens on a run."

Kim Draves describes herself as a get-off-the-couch runner. She used to run 3 or 4 miles every day and throw in a 10-K race every now and then to keep up her motivation. Then she had kids.

That was 11 years ago. Draves hadn't taken a step on the roads or inside a gym until January of 2011, when, filled with resolve, she made a commitment to become active again. She started morning workouts at the fitness center but couldn't get there consistently. "I needed flexibility," says Draves. "I needed something I could fit in every day even if only for 15 minutes. I wanted to keep on with my

plan to get fit, and running was the way."

So she stepped back onto the road, where she discovered a different obstacle. "It was so hard because of my frame of reference. I thought I'd just be able to go out and run, but I couldn't even do a mile," recalls Draves. "I couldn't breathe."

That spring, Draves signed on to Budd Coates's beginning running program. "The first day, we didn't even go outside," she said. "We lay on the floor learning to breathe." And that has made all the difference.

"I now have a tool that allows me to recover if I go out too fast or if something goofy happens on a run," says Draves.

"One morning I was running and I heard something coming up from behind. Then a guy on an ElliptiGO zipped past. It got me all flustered, but I told myself *count, breathe,* and it helped me recover and keep running. Before, I would have stopped and walked.

"On a long run, when it becomes more difficult toward the end, I focus on my breathing and the time goes by much faster," says Draves. "Running has become rhythmic, like a metronome." And Draves's consistent rhythm has made her the perfect long-run companion for her husband, who appreciates that Kim keeps his pace under control, too.

In the year and a half that Draves has been using rhythmic breathing, she's become faster and continues to improve. She has set her sights on a half-marathon, confident that with the control she now has over her breathing and pace, she'll be able to run consistently from start to finish.

CHAPTER 14

STRENGTH TRAINING

"You only ever grow as a human being if you're outside your comfort zone."—Percy Cerutty

T hough my belief in the value of strength training for runners hasn't changed in more than 30 years, the type of strength training I, and most experts, recommend has changed. Running requires specific work from the muscles in your legs and hips to move your body in one direction—forward. But your core muscles also play a significant role. They create stability and hold your body in good posture, from your lower back to your upper body. In addition, a strong core allows your breathing muscles to work more efficiently. The best strength program for runners includes exercises that will complement the muscles used in running and tone the core.

The other change I've made is in the way the individual exercises are done. For years I practiced and taught a circuit routine for runners that was based predominantly on resistance-training machines—it was safe and convenient and it increased strength. But the ideal way to train muscles for any activity is with exercises that most closely mimic the way you actually use those muscles—functional strength training. You exercise the whole movement rather than focus on individual muscles, because that's how your brain works—it directs full motion. Exercises performed with resistance machines tend to target individual muscles or groups of muscles rather than strengthen a full movement. Here's an example from everyday living: Squats performed with just your body weight or with free weights are more effective than a leg press at building strength for getting up from the couch—to go run.

There are many functional strength programs available, but assuming that running takes first priority, choose a routine that best complements the strength needs of a distance runner. My motto is "Lift to run; don't lift to get strong." Of course, you want to and will get stronger by lifting but in ways that apply to and improve your running. These two principles—strength for better running, functional training—are what guided the development of the program I recommend here for strengthening the muscles that make running more efficient. And I've added a new piece to the strength-training prescription for runners: exercises for your breathing muscles.

Strengthening Your Respiratory Muscles

Most of us don't even think about our diaphragms, let alone realize that it's a muscle we can strengthen. But rhythmic breathing, with its emphasis on diaphragmatic breathing, draws our attention to this large and essential muscle as well as to all of the muscles associated with the mechanics of respiration. Strengthening these muscles can increase lung volume, improve breathing efficiency, and enhance running performance in both training and racing.

Exercises that train your diaphragm and other inspiratory muscles through their full range of motion open the thoracic cavity to its maximum as you breathe. The larger the thoracic cavity, the more your lungs will expand, and the more air you will inhale. In addition, stronger respiratory muscles work more efficiently and take longer to fatigue, which makes breathing more efficient.

And the benefits don't stop there. As we discussed in Chapter 3, respiratory muscles take priority over skeletal muscle in the need for oxygen, so when your breathing muscles begin to fatigue, your central nervous system takes over and diverts blood (carrying oxygen) away from your legs to your respiratory muscles. Stronger breathing muscles take longer to fatigue, allowing a higher volume of bloodflow to your legs for a longer period of time.

You can strengthen your diaphragm (called inspiratory muscle training or IMT) while running at any level of fitness. For the beginning

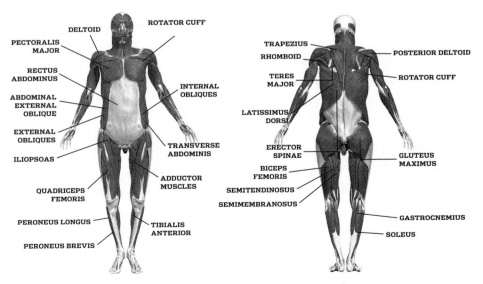

The muscles strengthened by the exercises in this chapter.

runner, merely learning to breathe diaphragmatically and then running at a 51 RBE will work the diaphragm more than it has ever been worked before. That stress, followed by a recovery period, helps strengthen this major breathing muscle. For the more experienced runner, long runs, tempo runs, hill runs, and long intervals performed in the 52-31 RBE range force full contractions of the diaphragm muscle for longer periods of time. More full contractions per minute not only requires a more forceful contraction of the diaphragm when you inhale, it also demands that the muscles used during exhalation (the expiratory muscles) kick in and assist in pushing air out of the lungs as the diaphragm relaxes. This, again, creates a training effect, and the muscles will come back stronger after recovery.

Training Underwater

Swimmers have learned how to add resistance to the action of breathing, which makes breathing more difficult and forces the diaphragm to work harder and, in time, get stronger. They do this using a snorkel equipped with an attachment that decreases the opening of the snorkel (the Cardio Cap is one such device). As the opening gets smaller, the swimmer must contract the diaphragm more forcefully to open the thoracic cavity and pull air into the lungs. When the swimmer concentrates on a full inhalation, the diaphragm must work through a full range of motion. On the exhale, the expiratory muscles must work harder to help push air out of the lungs and they, too, become stronger over time. Runners who choose to cross-train with swimming can use a snorkel in this way to strengthen their respiratory muscles. The beauty of swimming with a snorkel is that it eliminates one of the most difficult components of swimming—the head-in/head-out rhythmic breathing component. The snorkel allows you to concentrate on the work of your respiratory muscles. If you choose to perform IMT as a cross-training workout in the pool, consider investing in a Finis Snorkel with Cardio Cap.

Through the Nose

Being the running geek that I am, I attempted to apply the swimmer's method of IMT to running. I purchased a half dozen breathing masks, and during a treadmill run I changed the size of the holes to create various degrees of resistance when breathing. Strange, yes. During one of these trials my son, Colin, came down into our basement to check his laundry, and when he looked at me he just shook his head and said, "You're nuts."

Though the breathing masks worked, it was a bit odd, and I realized that there was another way—breathing only through the nose. Now, at all other times when you are running, you should breathe through both your mouth and nose. The more channels you have for air to enter your body, the more air you inhale. But if the goal is to limit airflow, resulting in increased work for the respiratory muscles, simply close your mouth.

Well, not that simply. First, plan to do breathing workouts on your moderate training days. Over time, if you want, you can add them to your easy days as well. But just as athletes who train at altitude come down from altitude for their quality runs, you should not combine breath training with your quality workouts. (You always want to do quality training in optimal conditions to get the most benefit from it.) Head out easily on your moderate run, and once you are running comfortably at a 51 rhythmic breathing effort, try breathing through your nose only for 1 minute. If you begin to feel lightheaded, switch back to breathing through your nose and mouth. You may need to slow your pace a bit as well. Once you feel comfortable again, try breathing through your nose. Alternate breathing through your nose with breathing through both your nose and mouth as it feels comfortable. Increase the amount of time breathing nose-only from workout to workout until you can run most of the workout using nose-only breathing. Once comfortable with the nose breathing, you can include it in any easy or moderate run, but discontinue practicing it 2 to 3 weeks prior to your goal race.

Using Resistive Breathing Devices

Resistive breathing devices, which are a bit more sophisticated than my series of breathing masks, have also been developed for IMT. You can choose from two categories of devices. One, represented by the brand Expand-a-Lung, requires you to create the same level of force during both inhalation and exhalation. The other, represented by PowerLung, offers you the ability to work at different levels of resistance during inhalation and exhalation. The PowerLung allows you to change both the inhalation and exhalation resistances independently and also allows a wide range of resistances to match your fitness level. Either device will be effective initially, but the greater range of the PowerLung will serve you better as your fitness improves. POWERbreathe also offers a wide variety of resistive breathing devices for runners at every level.

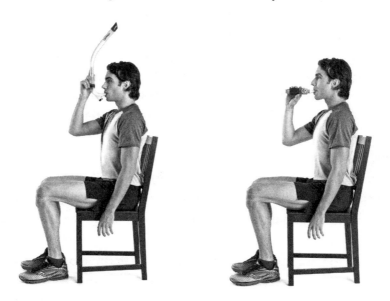

Finis Snorkel with Cardio Cap and PowerLung resistive breathing devices.

How best to use these devices to train your diaphragm? The thinking is that you can train the inspiratory muscles the same way that you train any working muscle. Most IMT devices come with exercise programs and recommend that you concentrate solely on diaphragmatic breathing when performing these exercises. I highly recommend adding a set or two during which you chest-breathe. This will force the intercostal muscles (both internal and external) of the chest to assist in inhalation and exhalation. During any physical activity, when your diaphragm begins to tire, your intercostal muscles will need to work harder. Train them now and reap the benefits later.

Core Training

Mention core exercises and most people will think of crunches, situps, and other moves that target the abdominal muscles, but in fact your core includes everything from your hips to your shoulders and connects your upper body to your lower body. Though the core itself does not perform any skilled technical movement in any sport, it's what enables the lower body and the upper body to do so. The core creates stability between the upper body and the lower body, allowing them to perform more effectively. In addition, the core muscles surround our vital organs, and the thoracic cavity and diaphragm rely heavily on the surrounding musculature for assistance and support.

A few years ago I developed a strength-training tool called the Core-Slider and, along with it, a series of exercises that enhance the strength of the entire core. Most every activity requires that you support your body in a specific position while you perform that activity. Running demands that you hold your body upright, push off leaving the ground, land on the ground, and repeat. The CoreSlider program works your core and upper body while requiring you to anchor yourself first from your knees and then from your feet as you advance in fitness.

As you do each exercise, you create a firm base with your lower body, forcing the core to work as a stabilizer so that your upper body can perform the movements in each exercise. When you perform this series of exercises using proper breathing, both your inspiratory and expiratory muscles work in unison with your core to open and close the thoracic cavity, training your respiratory muscles as well. You can find the CoreSlider online at TheCoreSlider.com.

The CoreSlider Workout

The exercises that follow are described as if you are on the face of a clock with your head at 12:00. Begin by warming up with stretching and do the exercises in the order given. Use a mat or some other cushioning to protect your knees.

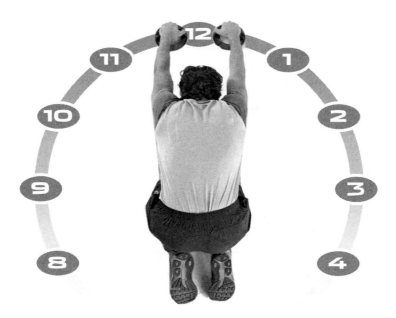

Starting positions.

Stretching Warmup

PART 1

1. Start in a kneeling position, hips on heels and CoreSliders at 12:00.

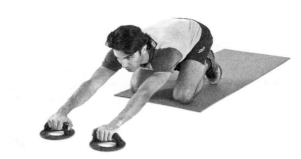

2. Keeping back and arms straight, lean forward as far as you can while pushing CoreSliders straight in front of you. Hold for 3–5 seconds. Return to starting position.

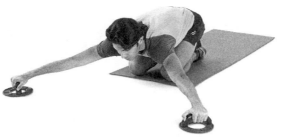

3. Gently push CoreSliders to 11:00/1:00 and hold for 3–5 seconds. Continue to 10:00/2:00 and then to 9:00/3:00, holding for 3–5 seconds each time and returning to start position between each.

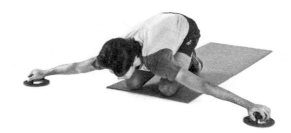

PART 2

1. Return to kneeling position, then push Core-Sliders to 12:00 and then in a wide circle down to your heels.

2. Circle CoreSliders back to 12:00 and return to starting position. Repeat 5 times.

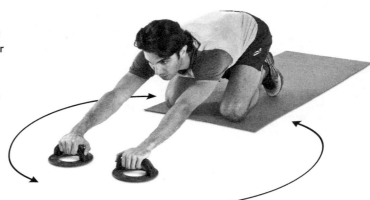

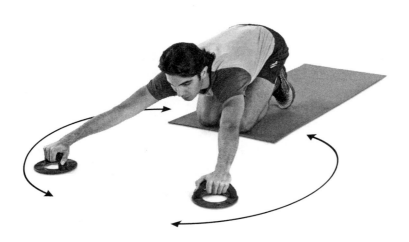

1. Pushups

1. Begin with the CoreSliders under your shoulders. Exhale.

2. Without moving the CoreSliders, inhale as you bend your arms at the elbow to 90 degrees and lower your torso toward the floor. Keep your upper body in a straight line.

3. Exhale as you return to the starting position. That's 1 rep. Pause and repeat 5–15 times.

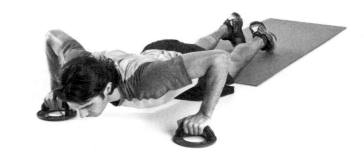

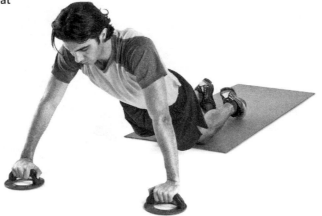

2. Double Time

1. From the starting position, inhale and push both CoreSliders to 12:00.

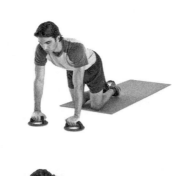

2. Exhale as you pull them back to center.

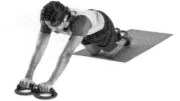

3. Next, simultaneously push the left CoreSlider to 11:00 and the right CoreSlider to 1:00 while inhaling. Exhale as you pull the CoreSliders back to center. Repeat (with breathing) at 10:00/2:00 and 9:00/3:00. May repeat 1–5 times.

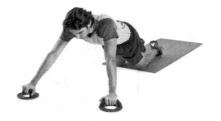

Note: You can also move to and from each clock position 1–5 times before moving to the next position.

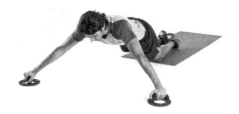

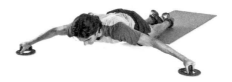

3. Wax On, Wax Off

1. Begin in the starting position with the CoreSliders under your shoulders.

2. Move each CoreSlider in an 18-inch circle going in opposite directions. (If you move the left one clockwise, move the right counter-clockwise.) Pull the CoreSliders back to the center as you return to the starting position. That's 1 rep. Repeat 5–15 times.

3. Repeat, this time reversing the direction of the CoreSliders, 5–15 times.

Note: To make the exercise more difficult, increase size of circles.

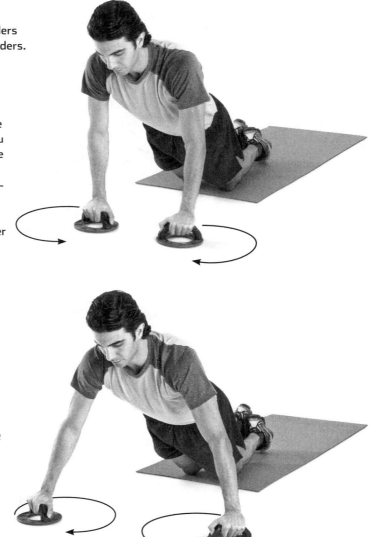

4. Fly Pushups

1. Begin in the starting position with the CoreSliders under your shoulders. Exhale.

2. While inhaling, keep the left CoreSlider still and bend your left arm at the elbow to 90 degrees as you slide the right CoreSlider to 12:00. Keep your upper body in a straight line.

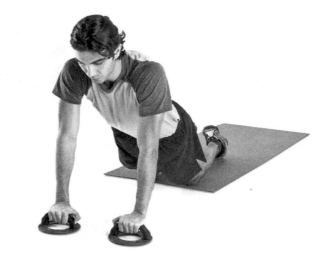

3. Exhale as you return to the starting position.

4. Repeat (using the same breathing pattern) while sliding the right CoreSlider to 1:00, then 2:00, then 3:00. That's 1 rep. Repeat 2–5 times. Repeat with opposite side.

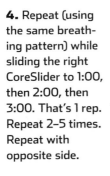

5. Plank

MOVE FROM the starting position into the final plank position by lifting your knees off the ground, moving your hips forward, and putting your weight on your hands and toes. Keep the CoreSliders below your shoulders. Hold for 5–30 seconds.

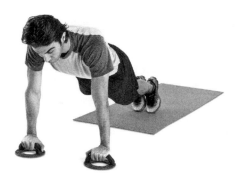

1. Rotate to the right and rise into a side plank position, keeping your right arm straight and resting your left hand on the left side of your abdomen. Hold for 5–30 seconds.

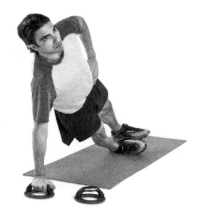

2. Sit down, then rise into a back plank. Hold for 5–30 seconds.

3. Sit down, then rotate left and rise into a second side plank position. Hold for 5–30 seconds.

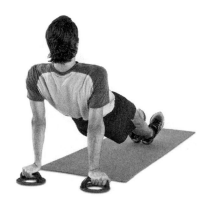

6. Assisted Situp

1. Sit at the back edge of the mat, legs straight, and CoreSliders at your sides. Exhale.

2. Inhale and, keeping your arms as straight as possible, push the CoreSliders to 9:00/3:00 as you lower your body, moving into a straight line from toes to shoulders and keeping your head slightly raised. Exhale as you return to the sitting position while pushing down on the CoreSliders. That's 1 rep. Repeat 5–15 times.

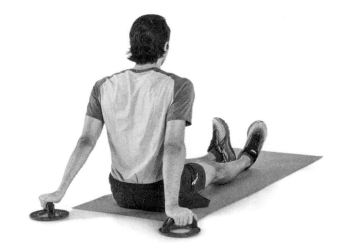

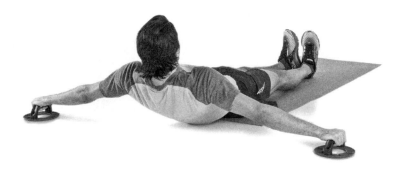

3. Repeat (using the same breathing pattern), this time pushing the CoreSliders back at an angle as you lower yourself; return to the sitting position for 1 rep. Repeat 5–15 times.

4. Repeat, pushing the CoreSliders back behind you as straight as possible; return to the sitting position for 1 rep. Repeat 5–15 times.

Note: Concentrate on using your arms more than your stomach muscles.

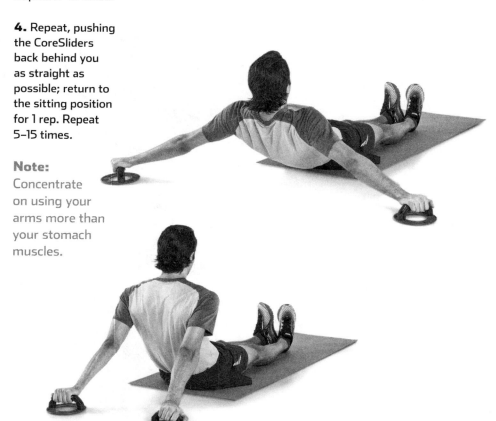

7. Straight–Leg Sitting Position

1. Begin by sitting with your legs straight. Cross your left foot over your right ankle, and rest the left CoreSlider on your stomach. Exhale.

2. Inhale as you lean to the right and slide the right CoreSlider out to the 3:00 position (your left hip may leave the floor). Exhale as you push downward with the right CoreSlider and return to upright position. That's 1 rep. Do 5–15 reps. Repeat at 9:00 on the opposite side.

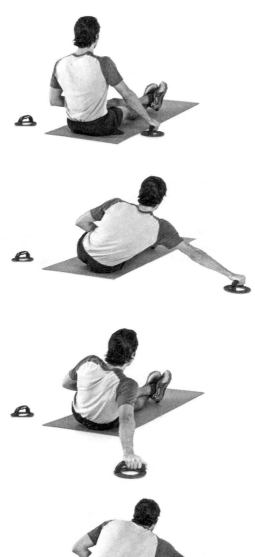

8. Roller Motion

1. Start in a kneeling position at the front of the mat, hips on heels, with the CoreSliders at 12:00. Exhale.

2. Keeping your arms straight, inhale as you move your hips forward as far as comfort allows and push the CoreSliders out, still at 12:00. Pause. Exhale as you return to hips on heels and bring the CoreSliders back to center.

3. Repeat (using the same breathing pattern), inhaling as you push the CoreSliders to 11:00/1:00 and exhaling as you return to hips on heels and bring the CoreSliders to center. Continue to 10:00/2:00 and to 9:00/3:00. That's 1 rep. Repeat 5–15 times.

Note: Change it up by doing reps at each position or in reverse.

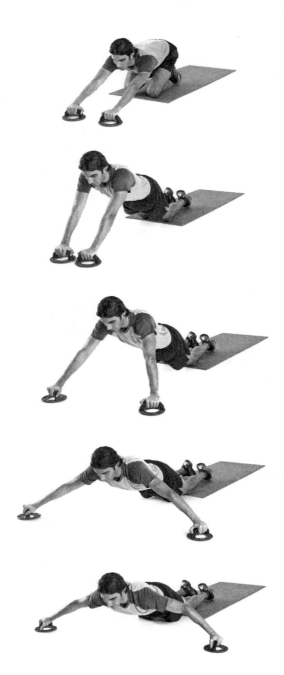

9. Reverse Snow Angels

1. Begin on your stomach with your arms next to your legs and hands in palms-down position. Push down on the CoreSliders for 1–3 seconds.

2. Begin moving the CoreSliders, pausing at 7:00/5:00 and pushing down for 1–3 seconds. Continue through each clock position until both Core-Sliders reach 12:00. Pause, then slide the CoreSliders back to the beginning position and exhale.

3. Next, inhale and push down on the CoreSliders as you circle up to 12:00; continue that pressure as you exhale and return to the start.

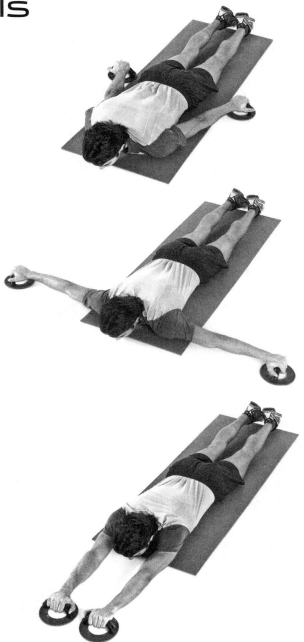

10. Snow Angels

Repeat exercise #9, this time lying on your back with your hands in the palms-up position.

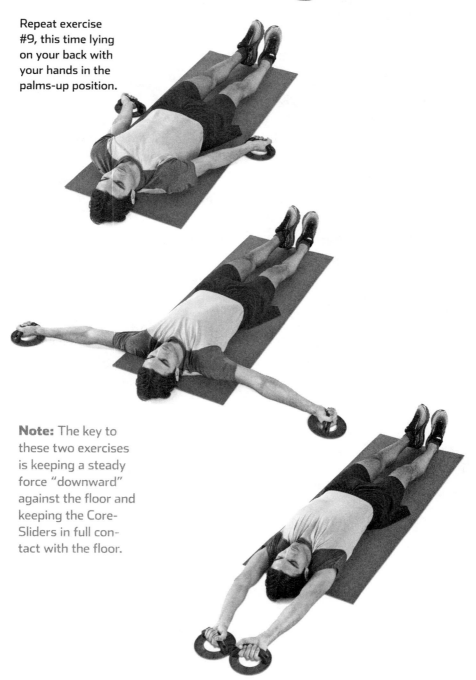

Note: The key to these two exercises is keeping a steady force "downward" against the floor and keeping the Core-Sliders in full contact with the floor.

Strength Training with Tubing

For those who do not own or have access to the CoreSlider, or who prefer working with resistance tubing, I've recommended an alternate program of 10 exercises using tubing that offers the same benefits to the core. This program can develop your stability to the point where you'll be able to stand comfortably on the rather unstable BOSU Balance Trainer, a device resembling a hemisphere that is used for balance training.

The tubing exercises shown below are more convenient and less expensive than free weights. Tubing comes in many tensions, denoted by color. Choose the tension that fatigues your muscles within the recommended 8 to 12 repetitions. When you can do 12 repetitions fairly easily, move up in resistance.

Perform the exercises in the order given for one full set and then repeat the full set two or three more times as desired. Specific breathing information is included with each exercise to most efficiently coordinate your inspiratory muscles with the exercise being performed. If you prefer to use Cybex or Nautilus equipment or free weights to do these exercises, alternatives to resistance tubing are given for each exercise.

1. Front Lat Pulldown

(alternative: lat pulldown machine)

Muscles trained: latissimus dorsi (lats), biceps, and rhomboids

DOOR STRAP
POSITION: high

STARTING POSITION:
Kneel, facing the door. Grasp one handle in each hand. Straighten your arms from your shoulders toward the top of the door. Slide away from the door to create tension (if necessary). Exhale fully.

1. Inhale as you bend your elbows and pull your hands to just outside your shoulders, pulling your shoulder blades together.

2. Exhale as you return to the starting position.

Repeat 8–12 times.

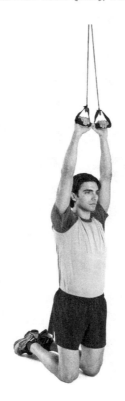
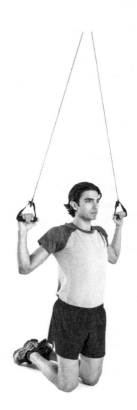

2. Arm Curl
(alternatives: arm curl machine or dumbbells)

Muscles trained: biceps

STARTING POSITION: Stand with your feet together. Grasp one handle in each hand and place the middle of the tubing under your feet. Inhale fully.

1. Exhale as you bend your right elbow and rotate your hand to face your shoulders.

2. Inhale as you return to the starting position.

Repeat 8–12 times, then switch to your left arm. (You can also work both arms simultaneously.)

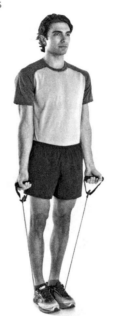

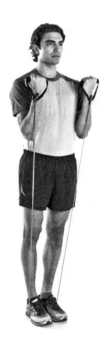

3. Standing Row
(alternatives: low-pull machine or dumbbells)

Muscles trained: latissimus dorsi (lats), biceps, deltoids, and rhomboids

DOOR STRAP
POSITION: waist high

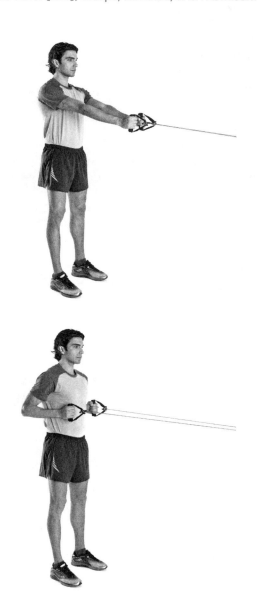

STARTING POSITION: Stand facing the door. Grasp one handle in each hand, palms facing each other. Step away from the door to create tension (if necessary). Exhale fully.

1. Inhale as you bend your elbows and pull your hands toward your stomach while pulling your shoulder blades together. Try to keep the tubing parallel to the floor.

2. Exhale as you return to the starting position.

Repeat 8–12 times.

4. Back Extension

Muscles trained: thoracic muscles and trapezius

**STARTING
POSITION:**
Lie on your
stomach with your
hands behind your
back and feet flat
on the floor. You
may need to have
a partner hold your
feet or position
them under a chair
to keep them from
coming off the
floor. Exhale fully.

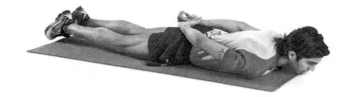

1. As you inhale,
raise your head
and shoulders off
the floor while
pulling your
shoulder blades
together.

2. Exhale as you
return to the
starting position.

Repeat 8–12 times.

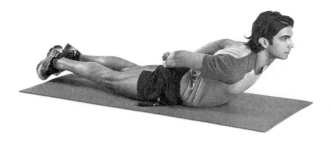

5. Bent–Arm Lateral Raise

(alternatives: lateral raise machine or dumbbells)

Muscles trained: deltoids

STARTING POSITION:
Stand with your feet together. Grasp one handle in each hand and place the middle of the tubing under your feet. Bend your elbows to 90 degrees. Exhale fully.

1. Inhale as you raise your elbows to shoulder level, keeping your hands in line with your elbows.

2. Exhale as you return to the starting position.

Repeat 8–12 times.

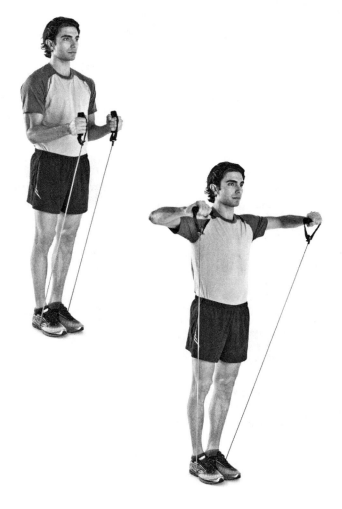

6. Side Chops
(alternative: high-pull machine)

Muscles trained: latissimus dorsi (lats), deltoids, and teres major

DOOR STRAP POSITION: high

STARTING POSITION:
Stand with your right side facing the door and your left foot about 2 feet behind you as shown. Hold the handles together using both hands. Extend your arms to the right, up, and toward the door strap. Move far enough away from the door to create tension. Inhale fully.

1. Exhale as you rotate your chest and shoulders away from the door and your arms down and to the left.

2. Inhale as you return to the starting position.

Repeat 8–12 times. Then repeat on opposite side.

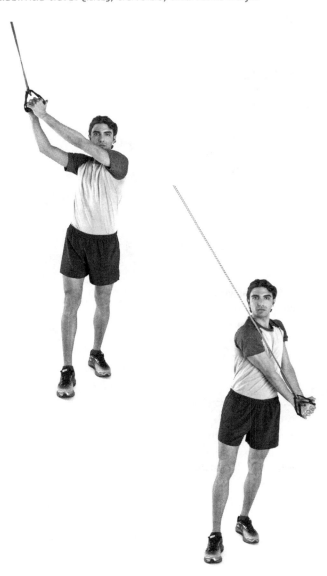

7. Pullover
(alternatives: pullover machine or dumbbells)

Muscles trained: latissimus dorsi (lats), abdominals, and pectorals

DOOR STRAP
POSITION: high

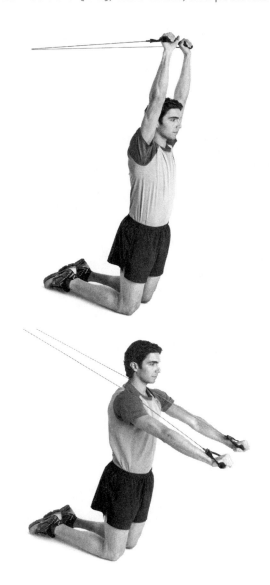

STARTING POSITION:
Kneel on both knees, facing away from the door, and grasp one handle in each hand. Slide away from the door far enough to create tension in the tubing, with your arms extended above your head and back as shown. Inhale fully.

1. Exhale as you rotate your arms forward and in front of your body, keeping your arms as straight as possible.

2. Inhale as you return to the starting position.

Repeat 8–12 times.

8. Fly Press
(alternatives: fly press machine or dumbbells)

Muscles trained: pectorals

DOOR STRAP
POSITION: chest high

STARTING POSITION:
Face away from the door. Grasp one handle in each hand and extend your arms forward at chest level. Exhale fully.

1. Inhale as you open your arms, like wings, to a full stretch.

2. Exhale as you return to the starting position.

Repeat 8–12 times.

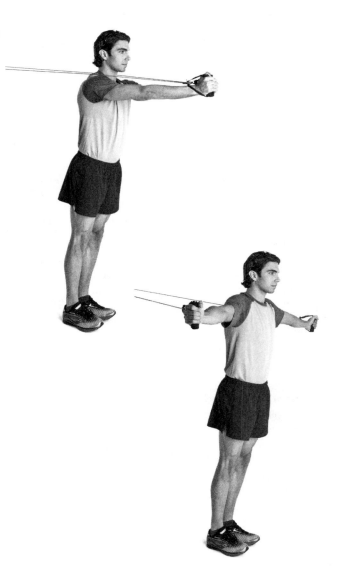

9. Triceps Press
(alternatives: triceps pushdown machine or dumbbells)

Muscles trained: triceps

DOOR STRAP POSITION: high

STARTING POSITION:
Face away from the door. Grasp one handle in each hand. Begin with your elbows bent, hands near your ears, palms up, and upper arms extended forward as shown. Inhale fully.

1. Exhale as you extend your arms forward to a straight position.

2. Inhale as you return to the starting position.

Repeat 8–12 times.

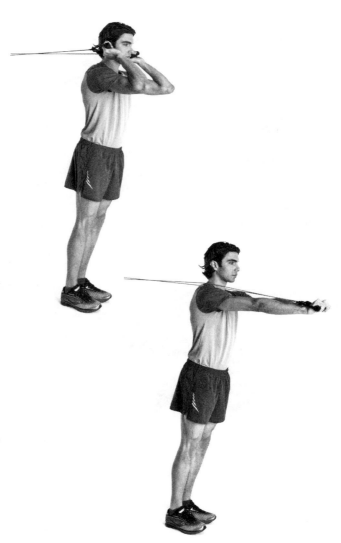

10. Plank

Muscles trained: erector spinae, rectus and transverse abdominis, glutes, and obliques

1. Lie facedown with your elbows and forearms under your chest as shown.

2. Push your body up off the floor, with your body in a straight line from your ankles through your hips and back to your shoulders (front plank). Hold this position for 3–5 seconds.

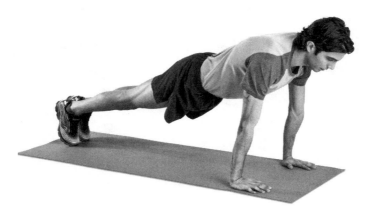

3. Lift your right arm off the ground and rotate your torso up and to the right with your right arm on your hip (side plank). Hold for 3–5 seconds.

4. Return to the front plank and hold for 3–5 seconds.

5. Flip over and perform the side plank to the left, holding for 3–5 seconds.

Repeat 5–10 times, alternating between left, front, and right side planks.

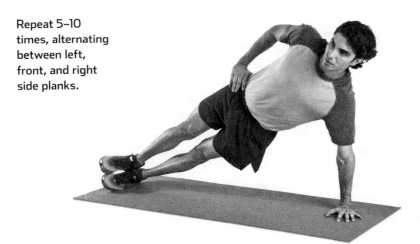

Rhythmic Runner:
Amy Weiss

RUNNER PROFILE: runs for fitness, health, and fun
AGE: 36
OCCUPATION: sales for a higher-education consultant

> "Rhythmic breathing makes running more comfortable, and I don't lose my breath anymore."

For cancer survivor Amy Weiss, breathing had once been her weakest link. "I'd run out of breath before my body would get tired," she says. After 2 years of treatments, first for lymphoma and then thyroid cancer, Weiss found herself starting all over again. She joined First Strides, a 12-week women's beginning running program, and at the end of the 12th week she could run a mile. Through First Strides, she signed up for a couple of Budd Coates's rhythmic breathing sessions, and that's when she learned how to hold on to her breath.

"Now I focus on my breathing when I run, and it helps me fall into a rhythm and pace that suits my level of ability," says Weiss. "Rhythmic breathing makes running more comfortable, and I don't lose my breath anymore."

What she *has* lost are the side-stickers that once would stop her in her tracks. She almost never gets them anymore, but if one should jab her, she knows what to do. "One day I was running with a group of friends and we were chattering away when we started up a hill. I found myself not only gasping for air but in pain, too," Weiss recalls. "I focused on my breathing and the side-sticker went away immediately."

Weiss is now running 3 miles four times a week and getting faster. She hopes to run under 30 minutes for a 5-K and maybe do a 10-K, too. Rhythmic breathing, you might say, has given Amy Weiss a second wind.

CHAPTER 15

STRETCHING

"The most beautiful motion is that which accomplishes the greatest results with the least amount of effort."—Plato

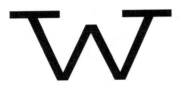hile suffering through my many injuries at Springfield College, I found that stretching before a run was not only painful but made my injuries worse. But stretching after a run felt more comfortable and seemed to help me rehabilitate from injury and prevent it. I decided to explore this in my master's thesis, "The Effect of a Post-Activity Flexibility Program on Muscle Soreness," at Illinois State University. Though the outcome of my research left me (and my advisor) with more questions than answers, the participants in the study were convinced that I was on to something.

Today athletes, coaches, physiologists, physiotherapists, massage therapists, yogis, athletic trainers, physical therapists, and sports doctors all

have varying opinions on stretching and whether or not it benefits the athlete. I've always believed that stretching is a necessary evil. Necessary because, if done correctly, it increases your range of motion. Evil because it takes time, almost always hurts, and can cause injury if done improperly. And static stretching before a race can slow the contraction rate of your muscles, which in turn produces a slow performance.

Yes, it takes time, which is probably the single most common excuse runners give for not stretching, but taking the time to stretch is worth every minute. Each of us has a natural stride length determined by the dimensions and mechanics of our bodies. Running regularly without stretching leads to a loss of flexibility and a loss of range of motion, which in turn shortens your natural stride length. It's generally been agreed upon that most runners have a stride cadence in the vicinity of 180 to 200 strides per minute, so you can see that the shorter your stride, the longer it will take you to run a given distance. That being said, the goal of stretching is *not* to try to increase your stride length but simply to allow your muscles unimpeded motion through your natural stride. With this comes less resistance and less chance of injury. Taking the time to stretch now means that you may not have to take more time later to recover from

Dynamic Stretching

What means of stretching could be more appealing than *dynamic* stretching, right? Dynamic stretching does have its role in the runner's bag of tricks, but it's a little tricky to execute. It uses sport-specific movements to prepare your body for that movement, and for runners that means leg or sprint drills. Done just before an interval workout or a race—after a 10- to 20-minute warmup run—it will actively increase your stride length, making a faster pace more comfortable.

But perfect form is important, so someone knowledgeable should teach you these drills and observe as you do them. Also, a dynamic stretching program should be built gradually into your training. Start with just a couple of exercises and add only one or two a week.

injury and regain your fitness. Stretching with the right method and at the right time—which I'll explain below—will prevent injury and allow you to progress toward your best performance. As for the pain...well, a good, healing deep-tissue massage hurts, too. And some will tell you it hurts so good.

Ways of Stretching

Over the years, many methods of stretching have been devised. You may remember old-fashioned ballistic stretching, during which the athlete used a "bouncing" movement to push the muscles beyond their range of motion. But when injuries resulted, this method was abandoned in favor of static stretching, in which you stretch the muscle to the point of tension and hold the stretch for 10 to 15 seconds (some suggest even longer). The drawback to the static method is that it can elicit the Golgi tendon reflex: When a muscle is stretched for too long, the Golgi tendon reflex kicks in and the muscle recoils in order to prevent tearing.

Along comes active isolated (AI) stretching. With AI stretching, you hold the stretch for only a few seconds to avoid the Golgi reflex. In addition, you contract the opposing muscle to let the muscle you are stretching relax and lengthen a little more. So, for example, to stretch your right hamstring (back of the thigh), you would lie on the floor and lift your right leg, forcing the quadriceps (front of the thigh) to contract; your hamstring relaxes so that the quadriceps can contract to lift your leg, and now you can stretch the hamstring a little more easily and a little farther.

There are other methods of stretching (see "Dynamic Stretching," opposite) and, as I've mentioned, everyone has an opinion on the best method. My experience as a longtime runner, coach, and fitness instructor has led me to recommend a combination of active isolated stretching and static stretching for the best and safest results.

When to Stretch

This also has evolved over time. Up until the '80s, experts and coaches recommended that you stretch as a warmup *before* exercise. But as researchers continued to study stretching, they learned that the best time to stretch is either after 10 minutes of aerobic exercise or after your workout. If you like to stretch at the beginning of a workout, ease into your run and after 10 minutes, if you have any sore areas, stop and stretch those areas specifically. Continue on your run and if that soreness persists, turn around and walk home. If you feel fine, keep running.

Before an interval session, it's helpful to perform a series of strides between your warmup and the start of your speedwork. This gradually increases your stride length—your active range of motion—and prepares you for the quicker-paced intervals. Light leg drills just prior to speedwork can further prepare your body for the work to be done, but make sure you know how to perform them correctly or have a coach oversee them. If, during the strides or drills, you notice any soreness, stretch those areas; if the soreness persists, bail on the workout.

Whether or not you stretch during the early part of your run, do so within 15 minutes of completing your workout—preferably after every run but definitely after every quality workout (intervals, hills, tempo, long runs). Quality runs cause the greatest fatigue, and fatigue causes muscles to become less flexible, which can make you more prone to injury. A regular postrun stretching routine will offset some—if not all—of this loss in flexibility.

The Stretches

I developed the following program around stretches for those muscles and muscle groups most affected by the stresses of running. Exercises that activate the gluteal muscles have garnered a lot of support recently, including mine. Activating these muscles, which two of these stretches do, enhances range of motion in the buttocks and hamstrings and increases performance.

The repeated segment of each exercise below uses AI stretching. Once the muscle or muscle group has adapted to the stretch so that the Golgi reflex will not be triggered, you can safely hold the position to finish. Use a stretching strap for optimal results.

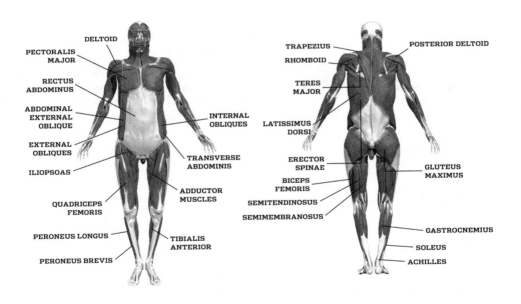

The muscles targeted in the stretches in this chapter.

Hamstring

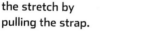

POSITION: Lie on your back, legs straight, strap around one foot. Then slide your free leg up to bent-knee position.

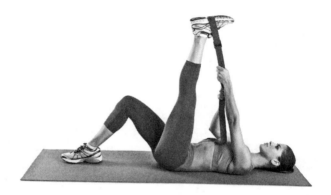

STRETCH: Contracting your abdominal muscles, hip flexors, and quadriceps, raise your straight leg up (knee locked) and toward your chest, bringing your leg as close to your chest as possible. Assist the stretch by pulling the strap.

HOLD: 3 seconds.

REPS: Repeat 6 times for a total of 7 reps.

FINISH: Repeat the stretch but hold for 18–20 seconds; then stretch the other leg.

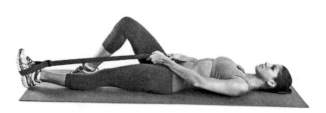

Adductors
(groin)

POSITION: Lie on your back, legs straight, strap around one foot.

STRETCH: Contracting the muscles on the outside of your hip, slide the leg with the strap out to the side. Assist the stretch by pulling the strap.

HOLD: 3 seconds.

REPS: Repeat 6 times for a total of 7 reps.

FINISH: Repeat the stretch but hold for 18–20 seconds; then stretch the other leg.

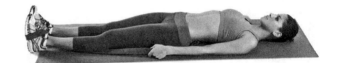

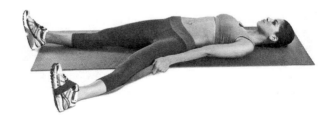

Abductors
(iliotibial band)

POSITION: Lie on your back, legs straight, strap around one foot.

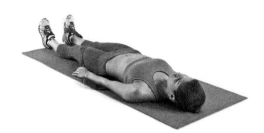

STRETCH: Contracting your abdominal muscles, hip flexors, and quadriceps, raise the leg with the strap (knee locked) as close to 90 degrees as possible. Keeping the knee locked, gently swing your leg across your body. Assist the stretch by pulling your leg down and to the side with the strap.

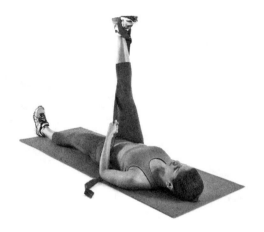

HOLD: 3 seconds.

REPS: Repeat 6 times for a total of 7 reps.

FINISH: Repeat the stretch but hold for 18–20 seconds; then stretch your other leg.

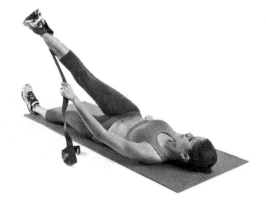

Hip Extension

POSITION: Lie on your stomach, legs straight, strap around one foot.

STRETCH: Bend the knee of the leg with the strap to 90 degrees and bring your arms over your head as shown. Contracting your lower back and gluteal muscles, raise the knee of your bent leg up off the ground. Assist the stretch by pulling the strap.

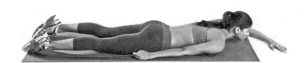

HOLD: 3 seconds.

REPS: Repeat 6 times for a total of 7 reps.

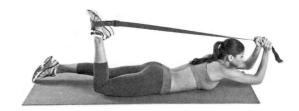

FINISH: Repeat the stretch but hold for 18–20 seconds; then stretch your other leg.

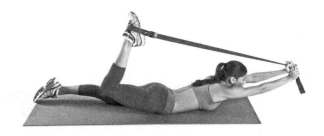

Psoas

POSITION: Kneel with one leg forward, foot flat on the floor.

STRETCH: Contracting your gluteal muscles, arch your back and move your hips toward your front foot. Do not allow one side of the pelvis to rotate in front of the other.

HOLD: 3 seconds.

REPS: Repeat 6 times for a total of 7 reps.

FINISH: Repeat the stretch but hold for 18–20 seconds; then stretch the other side.

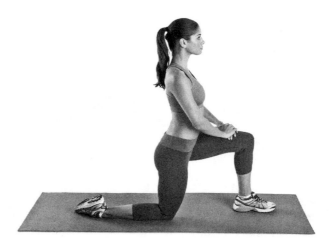

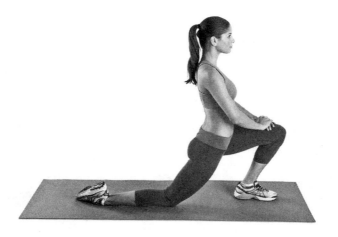

Pectorals

POSITION: Get
on all fours with
hands about 1 foot
forward from your
shoulders.

STRETCH: Slowly
move your hips
back and press
your chest and
shoulders toward
the floor while
contracting the
muscles in your
middle and
upper back.

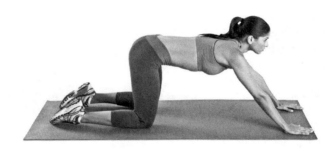

HOLD: 3 seconds.

REPS: Repeat 6
times for a total
of 7 reps.

FINISH: Repeat
the stretch
but hold for
18–20 seconds.

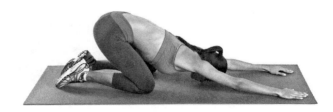

Calf

POSITION: Sit with legs straight in front of you, strap around one foot.

STRETCH: Contracting the muscle in your shin, flex your ankle to point your toe toward your body. Assist the stretch by pulling the strap.

HOLD: 3 seconds.

REPS: Repeat 6 times for a total of 7 reps.

FINISH: Repeat the stretch but hold for 18–20 seconds; then stretch the other leg.

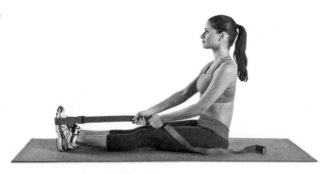

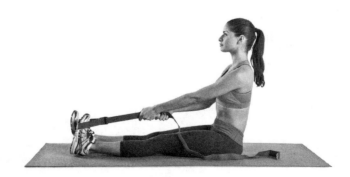

Achilles

POSITION:
Facing a wall or the back of a chair, stand a full arm's length away, hands pressed against the wall or holding on to the chair.

STRETCH: Raise your left heel off the ground; lean forward and, contracting the muscles in your shin, bend your right knee.

HOLD: 3 seconds.

REPS: Repeat 6 times for a total of 7 reps.

FINISH: Repeat the stretch but hold for 18–20 seconds; then stretch your other leg.

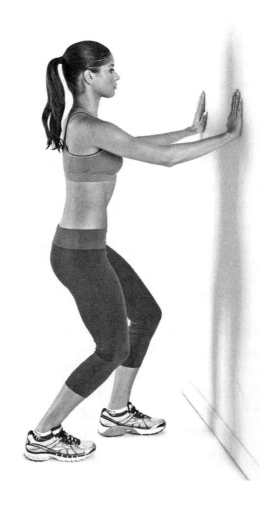

Acknowledgments

If you're reading this, I finally did it. Having worked at a publishing company for more than 30 years, I finally wrote a book. Well, that is, with the help and guidance of Claire Kowalchik. Thanks, Claire. And thanks to your two sons, Michael and Benjamin, for sharing their mom with me for 12 months. I would also like to thank my editor, Mark Weinstein. You read the manuscript with the eyes and insight that elevated this book to a new level. David Willey and John Atwood, I am grateful for your support and enthusiasm, which helped get the publication of this book rolling.

Running on Air has been more than 30 years in the making, and my wife, Ellen, has been there for me throughout most of those years. I met her at a race in the fall of 1981. She was running and I was watching. Thank you, Ellen, for welcoming generation after generation of running buddies to our home early on Sunday mornings and late Wednesday evenings as we trained for any number of races. Thank you for sharing miles of runs and races with me and now this book. Thanks also to our two children, Kelsey and Colin. In you we see ourselves and so much more.

Of course, this book has deep roots in my running history and the influence of those who introduced me to running and helped me along the way. I'll never forget our high school trip to States for cross-country in 1974, and I share that memory with Coach Vince Mellon and teammate Bruce Williams. I carry many great memories of my Springfield College teammates: Rick Cave, Jimmy Schlentz, Frank Young, David Van Houten, Jimmy O'Loughlin, W.F. New Hall III, and Scott Peterson. And it was during my years at Springfield that Dr. A.J. "Jack" Mahurin sparked my interest in the science of running and helped me find direction.

That direction led me to the many coaches and scientists mentioned and unmentioned in this book who have dedicated themselves to the sport of running and human performance. Through you I learned so much about training and physiology, and you inspired me to question and challenge popular concepts and philosophies. I hope this book does the same for you and generations of others.

Thank you, Dee Roberts and the late Bill "Coach" Coughlin, for being mentors in so many ways.

Bob Glover, you have an uncanny ability to always be wherever I need you to be: my first races at the Fish Hatchery 5-K in Rome, New York, and my first marathon in Miami, Florida, where you called me "Rookie," a nickname that you've used ever since. Thank you for cheering me on through 13 JPMorgan Corporate Challenge victories, for sharing one of the best "punks" in history with Coach Coughlin just days before we lost him, and for being an unyielding best friend.

Thanks to John Covert, my coach at Lehigh University, for your expertise and support. And to all my running buddies along the way, most importantly: Mark Will-Weber, Jim Knight, Fran Gough, Nip Brinker, Steve Sousa, Kenny Kunzman, Carl Kemerer, Lori Adams, Bill and Jane Serues, Mark Gerber, Todd Fach, Jamie Hibell, Shane Anthony, Kevin Sullivan, Robbie "the man" Patton, Joe McVeigh, Dan Gonzalez, Seth Kuchar, Kathleen and Mark Jobes, Rich Ryan, Bill Harris, and Craig Souders.

For those times when I didn't do it quite right and injured myself, I am grateful for the expertise and aid of Dr. Tom Dickson, Dr. Neal Kramer,

Dr. Frederick Jones, Dr. John Wolf, and Dr. Seith Schentzel, who got me back on my feet and running again.

With regard to the parallel path of my career, my gratitude goes out to those who pointed me in the right direction as well as the colleagues who have helped me enjoy a successful and meaningful experience at Rodale Inc. It was Jack Mahurin who led me to Dee, who introduced me to Dr. Charles Kuntzleman, who had enough faith in a young kid to recommend me for the employee fitness position at what was then Rodale Press. Thank you, Robert Rodale (former CEO) and Robert Teufel (former president), for seeing past the nervousness of that young kid and giving me the opportunity of a lifetime. Thanks to Pat Corpora, George Hirsch, Janet Glassman, Pat Richard, Joe Carter, Bob Kaslik, Mark Kern, Sue Weaver, Kate Delhagen, Mike Greehan, Pam Parker, Bart Yasso, Bob Wischnia, Amby Burfoot, Jane Hahn, Warren Greene, and many other Rodalians for sharing work, runs, and friendships. And, of course, to my excellent staff at the Energy Center (Rodale's employee fitness center), I appreciate your putting up with me all these years. Thank you, Maria Rodale, for believing in this company and its employees.

In conclusion, I go back to the beginning. I'm one of five children, three boys and two girls, who lost their dad at a very early age. I was 8 years old. My mother's job was difficult, but she persevered and, somehow, always saw the positive. Just a few years ago we lost my older brother, my younger brother, and my stepfather, but again, my mom found strength in herself and in her kids—me, Patsy, and Kathy—as well as her grandkids and great-grandkids. Mom, you've been an inspiration. And to my sister Kathy and brother-in-law Dave, thank you for your unwavering belief in me.

—Budd

Bibliography

Abraham, K. A., H. Feingold, D. D. Fuller, M. Jenkins, J. H. Mateika, and R. F. Fregosi. Respiratory-related activation of human abdominal muscles during exercise. *J Physiol*. 2002, Jun 1;541(Pt 2):653–63.

Albertus, Y., R. Tucker, A. St. Clair Gibson, E. V. Lambert, and D. B. Noakes. Effect of distance feedback on pacing strategy and perceived exertion during cycling. *Med Sci Sports Exerc*. 2005. 37(3):461–68.

Babcock, M. A., D. F. Pegelow, C. A. Harms, and J. A. Dempsey. Effects of respiratory muscle unloading on exercise-induced diaphragm fatigue. *J Appl Physiol*. 2002 Jul; 93(1):201–6.

Bailey, S. J., L. M. Romer, J. Kelly, D. P. Wilkerson, F. J. DiMenna, and A. M. Jones. Inspiratory muscle training enhances pulmonary O_2 uptake kinetics and high-intensity exercise tolerance in humans. *J Appl Physiol*. 2010. 109(2):457–68. Epub 2010 May 27.

Bonsignore, M. R., G. Morici, P. Abate, S. Romano, and G. Bonsignore. Ventilation and entrainment of breathing during cycling and running in triathletes. *Med Sci Sports Exerc*. 1998 Feb;30(2):239–45.

Boutellier, U., R. Büchel, A. Kundert, and C. Spengler. The respiratory system as an exercise limiting factor in normal trained subjects. *Eur J Appl Physiol Occup Physiol*. 1992;65(4):347–53.

Bramble, D. M., and D. R. Carrier. Running and breathing in mammals. *Science* 1983 Jan 21;219(4582):251–56.

Callegaro, C. C., J. P. Ribeiro, C. O. Tan, and J. A. Taylor. 2011. Attenuated inspiratory muscle metaboreflex in endurance-trained individuals. *Respir Physiol Neurobiol*. 2011 Jun 30;177(1):24–29. Epub 2011 Mar 5.

Carey, D. G., L. A. Schwarz, G. J. Pliego, and R. L. Raymond. Respiratory rate is a valid and reliable marker for the anaerobic threshold: Implications for measuring change in fitness. *J Sports Sci and Med*. Dec 2005(4) 482–88.

Downey, A. E., L. M. Chenoweth, D. K. Townsend, J. D. Ranum, C. S. Ferguson, and C. A. Harms. Effects of inspiratory muscle training on exercise responses in normoxia and hypoxia. *Respir Physiol Neurobiol*. 2007 May 14;156(2):137–46. Epub 2006 Sep 22.

Edwards, A. M., C. Wells, and R. Butterly. Concurrent inspiratory muscle and cardiovascular training differentially improves both perceptions of effort and 5000 m running performance compared with cardiovascular training alone. *Br J Sports Med*. 2008 Oct;42(10):823–27. Epub 2008 Feb 28.

Elkins, M.R., and J. D. Brannan. Warm-up exercise can reduce exercise-induced bronchoconstriction. *Br J Sports Med*. 2012 Oct 4. [Epub ahead of print]

Eston, R. Use of ratings of perceived exertion in sports. *Int J Sports Physiol and Perf.* 2012. 7:175–82.

Foster, C., K. J. Hendrickson, K. Peyer, B. Reiner, J. J. deKoning, A. Lucia, R. A. Battista, F. J. Hettinga, J. P. Porcari, and G. Wright. Pattern of developing the performance template. *Br J Sports Med.* 2009. 43(10):765–69. Epub 2009 Jan 5.

Girodo, M., K. A. Ekstrand and G. J. Metivier. Deep diaphragmatic breathing: Rehabilitation exercises for the asthmatic patient. *Arch Phys Med Rehabil.* 1992 Aug; 73(8):717–20.

Gontang, O. Give me oxygen and give me breath. *Mindfulness.* 2009 Jan 27. http://mindfulness .com/2009/01/27/give-me-oxygen-and-give-me-breath.

Green, J. M., A. L. Sapp, R. C. Pritchett, and P. A. Bishop. Pacing accuracy in collegiate and recreational runners. *Eur J Appl Physiol.* 2010 Feb;108(3):567–72. Epub 2009 Oct 29.

Gudjonsdottir, M., L. Appendini, P. Baderna, A. Purro, A. Patessio, G. Vilianis, M. Pastorelli, S. B. Sigurdsson, and C. F. Donner. Diaphragm fatigue during exercise at high altitude: The role of hypoxia and workload. *Eur Respir J.* 2001. 17(4):674–80.

Guenette, J. A., L. M. Romer, J. S. Querido, R. Chua, N. D. Eves, J. D. Road, D. C. McKenzie, and A. W. Sheel. Sex differences in exercise-induced diaphragmatic fatigue in endurance-trained athletes. *J Appl Physiol.* 2010 Jul;109(1):35–46. Epub 2010 Apr 22.

Guenette, J. A., and A. W. Sheel. Physiological consequences of a high work of breathing during heavy exercise in humans. *J Sci Med Sport.* 2007 Dec;10(6):341–50. Epub 2007 Apr 5.

Guenette, J. A., J. D. Witt, D. C. McKenzie, and J. D. Road. Respiratory mechanics during exercise in endurance-trained men and women. *J Physiol.* 2007 Jun 15;581(Pt 3):1309–22. Published online 2007 April 5. doi: 10.1113/jphysiol.2006.126466. PMCID: PMC 2170830.

Hatfield, B. D., T. W. Spalding, D. L. Santa Maria, S. W. Porges, J. T. Potts, E. A. Byrne, E. B. Brody, and A. D. Mahon. Respiratory sinus arrhythmia during exercise in aerobically trained and untrained men. *Med Sci Sports Exerc.* 1998 Feb;30(2):206–14.

Hill, A. R., J. M. Adams, B. E. Parker, and D. F. Rochester. Short-term entrainment of ventilation to the walking cycle in humans. *J Appl Physiol.* 1988 Aug 1;65(2): 570–78.

Illi, S. K., U. Held, I. Frank, and C. M. Spengler. Effect of respiratory muscle training on exercise performance in healthy individuals: A systematic review and meta-analysis. *Sports Med.* 2012 Aug 1;42(8):707–24. doi: 10.2165/11631670-000000000-00000.

Inbar, O., P. Weiner, Y. Azgad, A. Rotstein, and Y. Weinstein. Specific inspiratory muscle training in well-trained endurance athletes. *Med Sci Sports Exerc.* 2000 Jul; 32(7):1233–37.

Johnson, B. D., E. A. Aaron, M. A. Babcock, and J. A. Dempsey. Respiratory muscle fatigue during exercise: Implications for performance. *Med Sci Sports Exerc.* 1996 Sep; 28(9):1129–37.

Johnson, B. D., M. A. Babcock, O. E. Suman, and J. A. Dempsey. Exercise-induced diaphragmatic fatigue in healthy humans. *J Physiol.* 1993 Jan;460:385–405.

Kalsås, K., and E. Thorsen. Breathing patterns during progressive incremental cycle and treadmill exercise are different. *Clin Physiol Funct Imaging.* 2009;29(5):335–38. Epub 2009 Apr 22.

Kilding, A. E., S. Brown, and A. K. McConnell. Inspiratory muscle training improves 100 and 200 m swimming performance. *Eur J Appl Physiol.* 2010 Feb;108(3):505–11. Epub 2009 Oct 16.

Lima, E. V., W. L. Lima, A. Nobre, A. M. dos Santos, L. M. Brito, and R. Costa Mdo. Inspiratory muscle training and respiratory exercises in children with asthma. *J Bras Pneumol.* 2008 Aug;34(8):552–58.

Lomax, M., I. Grant, and J. Corbett. Inspiratory muscle warm-up and inspiratory muscle training: Separate and combined effects on intermittent running to exhaustion. *J Sports Sci.* 2011 Mar;29(6):563–69.

Lucas, S. R., and T. A. Platts-Mills. Physical activity and exercise in asthma: Relevance to etiology and treatment. *J Allergy Clin Immunol.* 2005 May;115(5):928–34.

Magness, S. Avoiding the hard/easy trap: Including moderate workouts can lead to outstanding results. 2010 Nov 2. http://runningtimes.com/Article.aspx?ArticleID=21097.

McMillan, G. Full spectrum lactate threshold training: Training to boost the top factor in performance. 2010 Dec 6. http://www.runnersworld.com/workouts/full-spectrum -lactate-threshold-training.

————. Performance page: Finding your sweet spot: Maximal vs. optimal adaptation rate. 2010 Nov 11. http://www.runningtimes.com/Article.aspx?ArticleID=21170.

Mickleborough, T. D., J. M. Stager, K. Chatham, M. R. Lindley, and A. A. Ionescu. Pulmonary adaptations to swim and inspiratory muscle training. *Eur J Appl Physiol.* 2008 Aug;103(6):635–46. Epub 2008 May 14.

Noakes, T. D. Fatigue is a brain-derived emotion that regulates the exercise behavior to ensure the protection of whole body homeostasis. *Front Physiol.* 2012;3:82. Epub 2012 Apr 11.

Noakes, T. D., J. E. Peltonen, and H. K. Rusko. Evidence that a central governor regulates exercise performance during acute hypoxia and hyperoxia. *J Exp Biol.* 2001 Sep; 204(Pt 18):3225–34.

Novotny, S., and L. Kravitz. The science of breathing. *IDEA Fitness Journal.* 2007;4(2): 36–43.

Quinn, T. J., and B. A. Coons. The talk test and its relationship with the ventilatory and lactate thresholds. *J Sports Sci.* 2011 Aug;29(11):1175–82. Epub 2011 Aug 21.

Romer, L. M., and M. I. Polkey. Exercise-induced respiratory muscle fatigue: Implications for performance. *J Appl Physiol.* 2008 Mar;104(3):879–88. Epub 2007 Dec 20.

Scano, G., M. Grazzini, L. Stendardi, and F. Gigliotti. Respiratory muscle energetics during exercise in healthy subjects and patients with COPD. *Respir Med.* 2006 Nov; 100(11):1896–1906. Epub 2006 May 4.

Scherr, J., B. Wolfarth, J. W. Christle, A. Pressler, S. Wagenpfeil, and M. Halle. Associations between Borg's rating of perceived exertion and physiological measures of exercise intensity. *Eur J Appl Physiol.* 2013 Jan;113(1):147–55. Epub 2012 May 22.

Shaw, B. S., and I. Shaw. Pulmonary function and abdominal and thoracic kinematic changes following aerobic and inspiratory resistive diaphragmatic breathing training in asthmatics. *Lung* 2011 Apr;189(2):131–39. Epub 2011 Feb 12. PMID: 21318637.

Simons, S. M., MD, FACSM, and G. G. Shaskan, MD. Gastrointestinal problems in distance running. *Int SportMed J*, 2005. 6(3):162–70. http://www.ismj.com.

Stickland, M. K., B. H. Rowe, C. H. Spooner, B. Vandermeer, D. M. Dryden. Effect of warm-up exercise on exercise-induced bronchoconstriction. *Med Sci Sports Exerc.* 2012 Mar;44(3):383–91.

Swart, J., R. P. Lamberts, M. I. Lambert, E. V. Lambert, R. W. Woolrich, S. Johnston, and T. D. Noakes. Exercising with reserve: Exercise regulation by perceived exertion in relation to duration of exercise and knowledge of endpoint. *Br J Sports Med.* 2009; 43(10):775–81. Epub 2009 Feb 11.

Tucker, R. The anticipatory regulation of performance: The physiological basis for pacing strategies and the development of a perception-based model for exercise performance. *Br J Sports Med.* 2009 Jun;43(6):392–400. Epub 2009 Feb 17.

Tucker, R., and T. D. Noakes. The physiological regulation of pacing strategy during exercise: A critical review. *Br J Sports Med.* 2009 Jun; 43(6):e1. Epub 2009 Feb 17.

Turner, L. A., T. D. Mickleborough, A. K. McConnell, J. M. Stager, S. Tecklenburg-Lund, and M. R. Lindley. Effect of inspiratory muscle training on exercise tolerance in asthmatic individuals. *Med Sci Sports Exerc.* 2011 Nov;43(11):2031–38.

Turner, L. A., S. L. Tecklenburg-Lund, R. F. Chapman, J. M. Stager, D. P. Wilhite, and T. D. Mickleborough. Inspiratory muscle training lowers the oxygen cost of voluntary hyperpnea. *J Appl Physiol.* 2012 Jan;112(1):127–34. Epub 2011 Oct 6.

Verges, S., O. Lenherr, A. C. Haner, C. Schulz, and C. M. Spengler. Increased fatigue resistance of respiratory muscles during exercise after respiratory muscle endurance training. *Am J Physiol Regul Integr Comp Physiol.* 2007 Mar;292(3):R1246–53. Epub 2006 Oct 26.

Vogiatzis, I., D. Athanasopoulos, R. Boushel, J. A. Guenette, M. Koskolou, M. Vasilopou-lou, H. Wagner, C. Roussos, P. D. Wagner, and S. Zakynthinos. Contribution of respiratory muscle blood flow to exercise-induced diaphragmatic fatigue in trained cyclists. *J Physiol.* 2008 Nov 15;586(Pt 22):5575–87. Epub 2008 Oct 2.

Vogiatzis, I., O. Georgiadou, I. Giannopoulou, M. Koskolou, S. Zakynthinos, K. Kostikas, E. Kosmas, H. Wagner, E. Peraki, A. Koutsoukou, N. Koulouris, P. D. Wagner, and C. Rous-sos. Effects of exercise-induced arterial hypoxaemia and work rate on diaphragmatic fatigue in highly trained endurance athletes. *J Physiol.* 2006 Apr 15;572(Pt 2):539–49. Epub 2006 Jan 26.

Vogiatzis, I., O. Georgiadou, M. Koskolou, D. Athanasopoulos, K. Kostikas, S. Golemati, H. Wagner, C. Roussos, P. D. Wagner, and S. Zakynthinos. Effects of hypoxia on diaphrag-matic fatigue in highly trained athletes. *J Physiol.* 2007 May 15;581(Pt 1):299–308. Epub 2007 Feb 22.

Wasserman, K., B. J. Whipp, S. N. Koyal, and W. L. Beaver. Anaerobic threshold and respi-ratory gas exchange during exercise. *J Appl Physiol.* 1973 Aug;35(2):236–43. PMID: 4723033.

Watsford, M. L., A. J. Murphy, and M. J. Pine. The effects of aging on respiratory muscle function and performance in older adults. *J Sci Med Sport.* 2007 Feb;10(1):36–44. Epub 2006 Jun 30.

Weiner, P., N. Berar-Yanay, A. Davidovich, R. Magadle, and M. Weiner. Specific inspiratory muscle training in patients with mild asthma with high consumption of inhaled beta2-agonists. *Chest* 2000 Mar;117(3):722–27.

Wells, G. D., M. Plyley, S. Thomas, L. Goodman, and J. Duffin. 2005. Effects of concurrent inspiratory and expiratory muscle training on respiratory and exercise performance in competitive swimmers. *Eur J Appl Physiol.* 2005 Aug;94(5–6):527–40. Epub 2005 Jun 8.

Whipp, B. J., and S. A. Ward. Determinants and control of breathing during muscular exercise. *Br J Sports Med.* 1998 Sep;32(3):199–211.

Witt, J. D., J. A. Guenette, J. L. Rupert, D. C. McKenzie, and A. W. Sheel. Inspiratory muscle training attenuates the human respiratory muscle metaboreflex. *J Physiol.* 2007 Nov 1;584(Pt 3):1019–28. Epub 2007 Sep 13. doi: 10.1113/jphysiol.2007. 140855. PMCID: PMC2277000.

Wyatt, F., L. Autrey, Y. Fitzgerald, S. Colson, and J. Heimda. Phase transition defines steady state beyond threshold. *J Ex Physiol.* 2004. 7(2); Epub 2004 Apr.

Suggested Reading

Astrand, Per-Olof, and Kaare Rodahl. 1977. *Textbook of Work Physiology*. McGraw-Hill.

Burfoot, Amby. 1997. *Runner's World Complete Book of Running*. Rodale Press.

Daniels, Jack. 2005. *Daniels' Running Formula*, Second Edition. Human Kinetics.

Daws, Ron. 1977. *The Self-Made Olympian*. World Publications.

Dreyer, Danny, and Katherine Dreyer. 2009. *Chi Running*. Fireside/Simon & Schuster.

Fitzgerald, Matt. 2010. *Run: The Mind-Body Method of Running by Feel*. Velo Press.

Glover, Bob, and Shelly-Lynn Florence Glover. 1999. *The Competitive Runner's Handbook*. Penguin Books.

Glover, Bob, and Jack Shepherd. 1977. *The Runner's Handbook*. Viking Penguin.

Higdon, Hal. 2011. *Marathon: The Ultimate Training Guide*. Rodale Books.

Lewis, Dennis. 1997. *The Tao of Natural Breathing*. Mountain Wind Publishing.

Liquori, Marty and Parker, John L. 1980. *Marty Liquori's Guide for the Elite Runner*. Playboy Press.

Livingston, Keith. 2009. *Healthy Intelligent Training*. Meyer & Meyer.

Lydiard, Arthur, and Garth Gilmour. 1978. *Running the Lydiard Way*. World Publications.

Martin, David, and Peter Coe. 1991. *Training Distance Runners*. Leisure Press/Human Kinetics.

McConnell, Alison. 2011. *Breathe Strong Perform Better*. Human Kinetics.

Miller, Thomas. 2002. *Programmed to Run*. Human Kinetics.

Mipham, Sakyoung. 2012. *Running with the Mind of Meditation*. Crown Publishing Group/Random House.

Mipham, Sakyong. 2003. *Turning the Mind into an Ally*. Penguin Group.

Murphy, Frank. 1992. *A Cold Clear Day*. Wind Sprint Press.

Myers, Larry. 1977. *Training with Cerutty*. World Publications.

Noakes, Tim. 2003. *Lore of Running*. Human Kinetics.

O'Brien, Justin. 2006. *Running & Breathing*. Yes International Publishers.

Romanos, Joseph. 1994. *Arthur's Boys*. Moa Beckett Publishers Limited.

Romanov, Nicholas, and John Robson. 2002. *Pose Method of Running*. Pose Tech Press.

Selye, Hans. 1978. *The Stress of Life*. McGraw-Hill.

Van Aaken, Ernst. 1976. *Van Aaken Method*. World Publications.

Wharton, Jim, and Phil Wharton. 1996. *The Whartons' Stretch Book*. TimesBooks/Random House.

Wilmore, Jack, David Costill, and Larry Kenney. 2008. *Physiology of Sport and Exercise*. Fourth Edition. Human Kinetics.

Index

Boldface page references indicate photographs and illustrations.
Underscored references indicate boxed text.

About the Authors

Budd Coates began running in 1972 at the age of 15, and 41 years later he can still run within seconds of personal bests set in his high school days. A student of running, coaching, and the science of the sport led him to a BS degree from Springfield College in 1979 and an MS degree from Illinois State University in 1980.

As the senior director of health and fitness at Rodale Inc., he has worked for the past 30 years with employees young and "not so young" to improve their health and fitness. An inventor, Budd has patents on The Bike Coach (a tool to help teach children how to ride a bike without training wheels) and The CoreSlider (a core and upper-body exercise tool). He has enjoyed an elite running career both in the US and internationally and has been honored as the JPMorgan Chase Athlete of the Year. Budd coaches beginner to elite runners and over the past 30 years of running and coaching has fine-tuned the content of this book, which he knows can change the way you run forever.

Budd lives in Emmaus, Pennsylvania, with his wife, Ellen; his daughter, Kelsey; and his son, Colin.

Claire Kowalchik has been running, writing, and editing for more than 20 years. She's completed countless road races and eight marathons, including twice running the Boston Marathon. Author of *The Complete Book of Running for Women*, she is also a former editor at *Runner's World* magazine and *Prevention Special Interest Publications* and is currently the editor-in-chief of *Diane*, a women's health and fitness publication from Curves International. She lives in Emmaus, Pennsylvania, with her sons, Michael and Benjamin Shimer.